Wakefield Press

Menopause

Menopause

Women tell their stories

Debra Vinecombe

Wakefield Press

Wakefield Press
1 The Parade West
Kent Town
South Australia 5067
www.wakefieldpress.com.au

First published 2008
Copyright © Debra Vinecombe, 2008
Copyright © individual contributors, 2008

Cover designed by Liz Nicholson, designBITE
Text designed and typeset by Clinton Ellicott, Wakefield Press
Printed in Australia by Griffin Press, Adelaide

National Library of Australia
Cataloguing-in-publication entry

Author: Vinecombe, Debra Constance, 1952–   .
Title: Menopause: women tell their stories/Debra Vinecombe.
ISBN: 978 1 86254 770 4 (pbk.).
Subjects: Menopause.
                 Middle aged women – Australia – Attitudes.
Dewey Number: 612.665.

For Sally

CONTENTS

A BEAR

In this life I'm a woman. In my next life, I'd like to come back
as a bear.
When you're a bear you get to hibernate.
You do nothing but sleep for six months.
I could deal with that.
Before you hibernate, you're supposed to eat yourself stupid.
I could deal with that.
When you're a girl bear, you birth your children
(who are the size of walnuts) while you're sleeping
and wake to partially grown, cute, cuddly cubs.
I could definitely deal with that.
If you're a mama bear, everyone knows you mean business.
You swat anyone who bothers your cubs.
If your cubs get out of line, you swat them too.
I could deal with that.
If you're a bear,
your mate EXPECTS you to wake up growling.
He EXPECTS that you have hairy legs and excess body fat.
Yup, gonna be a bear!

Author unknown

ACKNOWLEDGEMENTS

My deepest gratitude to the women who participated in this book, sharing their stories. My thanks to all the women who sent me letters and emails showing interest in the progress of the book and who continually encouraged me to see its completion. I also wish to thank the members of my writers group, Writers with Altitude, who have helped to make me a better writer, and to SA Writers' Centre for their resources and advice. Thank you to Lisa Marshall, photographer, and a very special thank you to Julia Wakefield for her creative cover ideas and for the many hours spent proof-reading. To my husband, Nigel, thank you for your support and belief in me to see the completion of this book.

FOREWORD

Menopause is tough. It rattles your mind, attacks your body, shakes your confidence and from time to time, as you sit in a puddle of sweat after another sleepless night, you wonder if you are going mad.

Debra Vinecombe's book spells out the facts, the myths and the day-to-day struggle of dealing with menopause in a compelling series of women's stories. I laughed. I cried. I was reminded of some of my worst times. And the funniest. Above all, I felt normal. Menopause may not affect us all the same way, but no woman escapes. It is a cycle. Bewildering and even frightening at times, but nevertheless a cycle.

In my mother's day, if menopause was discussed at all, it was in a whisper and delicately referred to as *change of life*. Now that I am almost through it (I hope!), I understand why. Your world spins and when it stops, you never find your old seat again.

Looking back, if I'd been armed with the information in this book from the start, the experience would have been much less fraught. I would have known precisely why I was feeling anxious, panicked, filled with despair, even dizzy, forgetful and nauseous. Menopause! Not madness. Not encroaching senility. Not a terrible illness.

Every woman should read these stories. So should her partner. Understanding what it's all about is the key to coping, overcoming and marching on to a new – but just as exciting – drumbeat.

Susan Duncan

Author of *Salvation Creek* (Random House)

INTRODUCTION

If you are a woman in your middle years, as I am, congratulations! You have either gone through menopause, are going through it now, or are about to experience it. We are lucky women. Few women around the late 1800s lived to reach the menopausal years. They died giving birth, from poor nutrition and disease, and from hard physical work. Those who did experience menopause sometimes found themselves locked away in the 'mad house'.

In the middle of the twentieth century, women had to endure their symptoms with little understanding or medical support, often feeling that they were indeed mad. Research on menopause continues today and it is still not known why the ovaries cease to function, bringing on menopause and all its associated changes. The mystery around menopause remains and when a woman experiences changes and feels anxious about this new stage in her life, she is sometimes reluctant to share her uncertainties.

It can be a busy time for a woman in her middle years. She's at the peak of her career or starting a new one, or she's retiring and planning a new direction. Her children may have left home, or returned home; perhaps she has no children either through choice or circumstance. She may have become a grandmother or is caring for her parents. She may be celebrating thirty years of marriage or perhaps her marriage is disintegrating; she may be alone or with a new partner. Whatever her circumstances, she is most likely unprepared for the changes that menopause can cause. She may associate a change to her menstrual cycle and hot flushes with menopause but she may experience other symptoms and be unaware of their association. Many women find menopause a bewildering, sometimes fearful, and lonely time.

It is often not until unexpected, perhaps severe, symptoms appear that a woman may go to bookstores or a library. She may log onto the Net, go into Google and type 'menopause'. A visit to her health practitioner may provide useful information and support but some women report dissatisfaction with traditional services. Hormone replacement therapy (HRT) and 'alternative' treatments are likely to be discussed and, depending on whom she talks to, one or the other recommended. Although a lot of the information is useful and interesting, it can be very clinical. Women feel that there is a gap in this information. A list of symptoms is a bit like a list of ingredients for a cake recipe but without the instructions. When I was going through my menopause I wanted to know what other women were feeling, how symptoms were affecting their everyday lives and what they were doing to manage menopause. I wanted real stories. I soon found out that I was not alone.

An idea for this book started to form. I placed advertisements in all states of Australia seeking women's stories. They came in the post and via email; I interviewed women in their homes or in mine and I talked to women for hours on the phone. Strangers were prepared to tell of one of the most difficult times of their lives. I discovered how distressing this time in a woman's life can be. I realised there was secrecy between women, and inconsistent and confusing information. I was surprised to learn that women who experienced the same symptoms and who managed those symptoms in the same way, could have very different outcomes. I included stories from women from all walks of life: varying ages, and different family situations, professions and interests; some have had serious health issues, others are in good health; and while some are going through menopause, others are post menopause.

This book has been written to connect women through their menopausal years. It gives information, support, comfort and understanding. In some cases the stories have been difficult to tell and the writing of them has been a journey in itself. Why? Western society does not make it easy to talk about how some symptoms of menopause can affect women. It is hard to talk about depression, panic attacks, incontinence, a dried-up vagina. It's difficult to get through each day confused and forgetful, trying to be nice yet feeling miserable, even hateful. And at night, getting up to change a sweat-soaked nightie for the third time and finding it impossible to sleep. Morning arrives, she is tired and vulnerable, fighting back tears. No one asks what's wrong. It's not talked about.

Well, no longer. This book *is* talking about menopause. It's talking about the denial; the ignorance and fear; the symptoms and menopause's impact on health, aging, career and relationships. It's exposing the secrets and mystery. The stories in this book go beyond the medical description of menopause, the list of symptoms and treatments. They connect women with real life stories.

Not all experiences are the same and not all symptoms will be relevant for every woman. However, all women undergo hormonal changes. The degree to which each woman's body responds to these normal hormonal changes varies. The intention of this book is not to promote nor detract from any particular therapies, be they HRT, natural or herbal. Nor does it advocate one method over another. There are already plenty of books and information available to cover these areas. However, in the following stories women do talk about their handling and management of symptoms, including medical and natural methods.

IN THE BEGINNING

Menopause means the last menstrual period. Perimenopause, which lasts two to six years on average but which can take ten years or even longer, is the time leading up to this last period when women usually experience symptoms of menopause. Menopause is the term commonly used to refer to the time both just before and after the last period, and occurs, on average, when a woman is in her mid forties to mid fifties. It is the time when the ovaries stop producing oestrogen and progesterone. It is usually a gradual process taking several years, but it can also occur suddenly for some women. Reduced oestrogen means physical and mental changes. In the beginning (the perimenopause stage) a woman notices a change to her menstrual cycle. The monthly period becomes erratic. It may become several days longer than usual, or shorter. A period may be missed for one month or several months and then it may return. The bleed may become heavier, or lighter. An irregular cycle may last for years before menstruation finally stops.

Hot flushes in the day and sweats at night are other early signs of menopause. Parts of the body feel hot, often burning hot, and sweaty. Commonly, night sweats disrupt a woman's sleeping pattern. She may find that she is constantly kicking off her bed covers to cool her overheated body, only to drag the blanket back on because of shivering cold. Getting out of bed to wash or change her bedding disturbs her sleep even more and after several nights of this, insomnia can set in. She will start the day feeling tired and perhaps her joints are stiff with pains in her hips and cramps in her legs. As the day progresses she may have difficulty in concentrating, remembering appointments, making decisions. At the end of the day she is understandably irritable, snappy and exhausted. The same disturbed night follows. This pattern can be devastating to a woman trying to perform her many daily duties.

For some women menopause starts earlier than the average age of forty-five, occasionally before the age of forty. Premature menopause will occur after surgical hysterectomy when both ovaries are removed, or it may be genetic or induced from radiotherapy or chemotherapy. Women who smoke tend to experience menopause around two years earlier than non smokers. Menopause as a result of surgery or medical treatment is often immediate with more severe symptoms.

Premature menopause can be very distressing for women who have not fulfilled their plans to have children. Because premature menopause is uncommon, symptoms may not be thought of as menopausal.

PSYCHOLOGICAL SYMPTOMS

With the many hormonal changes happening in a woman's body, psychological symptoms such as mood changes, sadness and tears, confusion and forgetfulness, anxiety and depression, can occur. Sometimes these symptoms can be attributed to insomnia or other stresses, but it is important that women who suffer from emotional or cognitive symptoms understand the possible connection to menopause and reduced oestrogen production. The knowledge that these symptoms might be experienced during menopause can help to alleviate anxiety and fear.

SEX

Oestrogen plays an important role in maintaining healthy vaginal tissue. In the late stages of menopause, when oestrogen levels have fallen significantly, the tissues that line the vagina and urethra become dry, thin and less elastic. A dry vagina causes irritation and discomfort and sex may be painful due to the lack of lubrication and reduced elasticity of the vaginal walls. A woman may be less interested in sex than she was pre-menopause. Not surprising if her vagina is dry and sore. In addition, a woman on average has only half the testosterone (sometimes referred to as the sex hormone) in her mid forties as she had in her twenties. The reduction of oestrogen and testosterone may directly affect libido and many women experience difficulty in achieving orgasm, or find that it takes longer and is less intense. Some women who have found intercourse too painful are satisfied with cuddles and kisses, closeness and companionship. On the other hand, they may be experiencing unusually sensitive skin or a prickling sensation (some have likened it to ants running over the skin) and cannot bear to be touched. Changes in the vagina, urethra and bladder at menopause can make women more susceptible to urinary tract infections. Other complaints include frequent and painful urination with a feeling of needing to urinate when the bladder is in fact empty. As the tissues of the vagina and urethra lose their elasticity and the pelvic floor muscles weaken, women may also experience urinary incontinence.

AGING

No one welcomes the signs of aging – female or male. Some signs we see every time we look in a mirror and others we feel. Unfortunately social attitudes in Western culture put more value on looking young and slim, with flawless skin and luscious hair. Billions of dollars are spent on age-defying products to keep the youthful look. However, as we age it is normal for our skin to become thinner and less elastic due in part to the reduction in oestrogen. Some women are lucky to have youthful-looking skin throughout menopause, but notice a change following menopause when the ovaries cease producing oestrogen. The skin may become drier or oilier; wrinkles increase; cuts and abrasions often take longer to heal; and bruising occurs more easily. Testosterone changes can cause an increase in facial hair, particularly around the jaw line, and thinning of hair on the head. Pubic hair also can thin. Although life-style practices such as diet and exercise play an important role in our body weight, some women experience a shift of body fat from the buttocks and legs to the abdomen area during menopause.

OSTEOPOROSIS

Osteoporosis is a condition in which bones become fragile, brittle and thin leading to an increased incidence of fractures, often after only a minor fall. The most common breaks occur in the hip, wrist and spine. There are many reasons for bone loss including a family history of osteoporosis, diet and lifestyle, certain medications and some health problems such as diabetes. Bone loss is accelerated at menopause due to the reduction in oestrogen and the most rapid bone loss occurs immediately after menopause. To assess whether osteoporosis is a risk factor, a health practitioner can arrange for a bone density scan to be done. This technology keeps a check on the progress of the disease and monitors the effects of any recommended treatments which may include prescribed medicines, as well as a diet rich in calcium, exercise and other lifestyle considerations.

SEEKING INFORMATION AND ADVICE

Whatever your experience of menopause I recommend that you use the internet and at the back of this book are useful contacts and web sites. The women's hospital in your capital city will also be able to direct you to appropriate contacts.

Discuss your menopause with health professionals: your local general practitioner and specialist (or two), naturopaths and herbalists, until you find someone with whom you feel completely comfortable. Talk about all your symptoms. Do not hold back. Ask questions about any proposed treatment, how it will help you, the risk factors and side effects, and the likely term of the treatment. Talk to your mother, girlfriends and your partner about your feelings and symptoms. If you are in a relationship it is a journey for two, not one.

Be kind to yourself. You are not falling apart, you are just going through some natural changes. Do not go through them alone. Share them, listen to advice and accept help. Women from all over Australia have shared their stories so that you may be able to relate to an experience and think, 'That is what's happening to me. I'm not going mad after all.'

DEBRA'S STORY

Ask my friends and family to describe me and they will use words such as organised, efficient, capable. At forty-nine I thought I'd had an easy time of menopause. Six months later my life was barely recognisable.

The real-estate agent looked through our house, room by room. Clipboard in hand, she ticked boxes – three bedrooms, study, new kitchen, no en suite (lost points here), pretty garden, ghastly shed, and so on. I followed her like a puppy. She said it would be no problem to sell but in order to get the maximum price she suggested a few improvements. I wrote them down, agreeing because we wanted top dollar. Then she gave me the names of people who could help: plasterer, painter, carpenter, gardener, cleaners, interior designer. Dates were set for open inspections and the auction. She was blonde and trendy, looked twenty-two but had the confidence of a thirty-year-old. I waved goodbye as she drove off in her new BMW. I walked indoors and looked around my spotless, shining, not-a-thing-out-of-place home. I looked at the list of jobs she had given me. Bloody cheek.

Before I got cracking on the house make-over, I saw my doctor for my two-year checkup: pap smear, blood pressure, cholesterol count, breast check. My periods had ceased about a year earlier when I was forty-eight. It was no drama; they just got lighter each month and then stopped. I didn't mourn the passing of my menses; I didn't feel any less of a woman or that I had lost a vital part of my femininity. I was glad to be rid of the backache, headaches, groin ache and stained clothes. I was enjoying the freedom. Menopause God bless you!

'Since my last visit, I've gone through menopause. Breezed through it,' I bragged, and told the doctor the date of my last period.

'You may still get symptoms,' she said. 'I think we'll take a blood sample so there's a record of your hormone levels.'

'Okay,' I agreed. 'So, menopause hasn't necessarily finished with me?'

'Maybe not,' and she slid the needle into my vein, filling the tube with cherry-red blood. I looked away, feeling faint.

'Come and see me if you have any problems.'

I wondered what problems there could be. But I had no time to think of it. I had a house to get ready for sale.

I stripped the paint off the window frames, sanded back and painted. Inside and out. I filled the cracks, sanded them smooth and painted walls, ceiling and cornices. The curtains were washed, pressed and rehung onto millions of tiny hooks. I thought an iron rod had replaced the bones in my neck. I scoured the bathroom tiles and regrouted the grout. I hooked the trailer onto the car, drove back and forth to the sand and metal place and shovelled tons of new white gravel onto the driveway. I painted the ghastly shed, roof too. I replaced the broken glass in the shed window, smashed so many times with the cricket ball, soccer ball, and just for the hell of it. I crossed off job number eighteen. Only fifty left to do!

I was tired but I wasn't sleeping well. It was the middle of winter and I was feeling too warm in bed. This was unusual for me. I really feel the cold. I normally sleep in a flannelette nightie under a quilt marked 'for blizzard conditions'. I wondered if I should turn the electric blanket off. I would stick my legs out to cool down but would quickly get cold. This continued and just when I needed a good night's sleep, I would lay wide awake. I couldn't switch off and started to become anxious. Anxiety was foreign to me. But I dismissed it, thinking, 'I've worked like a slave all day and have so much to do.'

The first open inspection was a week away. I spent several days redesigning and replanting the whole garden, colour covered the freshly turned soil and edges were sharply trimmed. Carpets were steam-cleaned and windows washed. Dust, polish, fluff up, plump, smooth out. Fresh flowers, fruit bowl (had to be a green bowl with oranges said the agent). Ready!

I did not feel my normal self but had to keep going. I was desperate for sleep but was too warm even after changing the bedding to summer conditions. I worked out that it must be hot flushes; the doctor had said I could expect menopause symptoms. But I was so anxious. Why? A friend said that I was doing too much. I knew that wasn't it. It was the fourth house I had prepared for sale and I was six months pregnant during the last one! Physical work was not alien to me, nor was being busy, juggling a dozen things at once. But something was not quite right. Was I missing my husband whose work had taken him overseas for a few weeks? No, I had always been fine in his absences.

Our son was at high school, doing well, no worries there. I was fit and healthy; it is part of who I am. In my twenties and thirties I was a qualified fitness instructor and personal trainer, not only taking aerobic classes but also teaching nutrition. So I knew how to look after myself. I kept going back to the question: Why am I feeling anxious? So anxious that I was concentrating to keep myself together. When I lay in bed I noticed that my heart seemed to be racing and I was breathing faster.

My husband returned to see a SOLD sticker on the billboard and his wife wafer thin. I am normally thin, but I had lost six kilograms and looked haggard. My eyelids hung in sagging folds, my vision down to narrow slits. Emotionally, I was in tatters, fighting back tears, struggling to understand what was happening. Was I losing it? I talked to myself sternly, disgusted with my weakness. Did anyone notice? Probably not. No one had ever had to worry about me. I was the planner, the organiser, the fixer, the reliable one.

Settlement was a month away and I started the tedious job of packing – ninety-three boxes! I organised a garage sale and the shed (not so ghastly now) was swept and decobwebbed and filled with rusting garden furniture, cracked pots, blunt tools, old bikes with punctured tyres – boxes and boxes of stuff. Treasure hunters arrived at five in the morning.

With an empty house, we moved to the Adelaide Hills where we have sixteen beautiful acres and a gorgeous cottage. We bought the land years ago and had planted an orchard and two acres of garden, erected three kilometres of fencing, cleared paddocks of blackberry and gorse and built our cottage. I love this place. Settlement was a few days away. All that was left was to clean the inside and mow the lawns. Then we handed over the keys.

It was evening. The ducks were squabbling down by the dam and the cows chewed the cud. We had just finished dinner.

'Could you mow the lawns at the house on Saturday please, Nige?' My husband groaned and asked why Saturday. I exploded with a fit of screams and tears.

'I'll do them, but one night after work,' he said, astounded at the hysterical vision in front of him. I ran into the bathroom, babbling and howling, unable to stop. Some minutes later I heard movement in the kitchen and water filling the sink, dishes being cleared from the table. Father and son agreed they ought to do something. My legs crumbled beneath me. A few minutes later I heard kind words, and strong hands lifted me from the floor and carried me onto the bed. I could not stop crying. Our son brought in a wet flannel and wiped my face.

'Okay, I'll mow the lawns on Saturday,' said Nigel gently, hoping this would calm me. In pidgin English I mumbled that something was wrong with me and I didn't know what. I was undressed and put into bed with a glass of water and two paracetamol. The following morning, Nigel took his first sick-leave day in twenty years and I was extremely grateful. He drove me to the doctor and we sat in her room as she listened to my tear-filled words. She took a blood sample and got the results immediately.

'No wonder you're feeling like this,' she shook her head. 'You've lost a bucket-load of oestrogen, Debra, since I saw you last.'

And that was how my menopause symptoms started. On earlier visits to my doctor, I made it clear that I didn't want hormone replacement therapy (HRT). There were several reasons for this. My fitness and nutrition training dictated a 'natural' lifestyle and I had always employed non-medical remedies for ailments in the first instance. Rest, water, fresh fruit juices, garlic, massage – simple things. If they didn't work, I had no problems with using medication after I asked a load of questions regarding side effects. I read books and pamphlets on HRT, the pros and cons, and on balance decided it was not for me. I attended a course, Menopause Naturally, and a lot of those suggestions did not convince me either.

But what to do? I clearly needed help and as my doctor knew my feelings on HRT, she suggested a course of Cipramil. She explained that I needed to kick-start the hormone serotonin in my brain, which she said was depleted. She likened the situation to driving a car and running out of petrol. I was strongly against this. Society attaches a terrible stigma to antidepressants. Furthermore, I said that I wasn't depressed. She looked at her notes – anxiety, heart palpitations, rapid breathing, insomnia, weight loss, crying. In summary, a miserable wreck. She gently placed the prescription in my hand and said to keep it, just in case.

I had hoped that now that I knew my symptoms were part of menopause, now that I had a name, an answer, I would manage. Mind over matter. I planned to make an appointment to see my friend Sue, a qualified herbalist. I would go to the library and borrow everything on menopause, get in touch with Women's Health Statewide and ask my best friend Gaye, who is a wiz on computers, to search the Net. I didn't last twenty-four hours. I couldn't even organise myself to get dressed, let alone do a research project. Something had shifted inside me. It would be too easy to say that it was all the work I had done to prepare our house for sale. I knew it wasn't that. I felt that I had lost all that had been me. After another sleepless night, full of worry, I said to Nigel, 'I have to get those pills.' He agreed.

The instructions said one pill three times a day. There was also a long sheet with about a hundred possible side effects, including death. But as I felt close to dying anyway, I took one pill a day. The effect was almost immediate and on the second day I felt fantastic. A human being again. I took a deep breath, as if it was my first in months. I had slept for a few hours and stopped crying. I felt some energy return. I was less fragile. After a week I was on a high. I was driving back from the shops, sunroof open, music playing loud and singing at the top of my voice. I unpacked the shopping, danced around the kitchen and thought, 'This feels great.' But I had enough sense to know that it wasn't normal.

I stopped taking the pills thinking that I was cured. The next morning I spent the day wandering around aimlessly in my dressing gown, full of fear. I reasoned that one pill a day had been too many, but none took me right back to hell. I worked out that one pill every other day kept me functioning well enough, although I still felt just below par. I kept this routine going for two months, then weaned myself off the following month, stopping altogether after three months. My doctor wasn't happy with my decision and talked to me again about taking a course of HRT. But I felt stable and promised her that I would come and see her immediately if I needed to.

I started my research. First stop, friends. I have a group of very close girlfriends whom I have known for over twenty years. We met through work and have kept in touch with a dinner every couple of months. We have supported each other through relationships, pregnancies and miscarriages, career changes and operations, and seen our children born and grow into adults. During one of our dinner evenings, I casually mentioned that I had lately had a distressing time with menopause. I was fishing. They, too, were going through the change and we all gingerly stepped around symptoms. By the end of the night all four of us had confessed to taking antidepressants to get us through a particularly bad time. One friend had taken a course two years earlier and kept it to herself because of the shame. We were all shocked that we had kept this from each other and pledged to be honest in the future, agreeing that emotional support was vitally important at this time in our lives. Amazingly, all of us admitted that we knew very little about menopause, despite being educated women.

Next stop was a visit to the Women's and Children's Hospital in Adelaide where I gathered many brochures, most of them produced by The Jean Hailes Foundation in Victoria. Gaye down-loaded pages and pages on menopause and I borrowed all the books available from the library. I also consulted Sue, my herbalist, who has known me for fifteen years. Sue is professional and thorough, and she regards each person as an individual. Genetic information, life story, diet, emotional and mental state, including a sense of purpose or connectedness to something – call it spirituality – all make up a picture of the individual for her. Therefore the 'remedy' she prescribes is different for each person, regardless if they present with the same symptoms. I explained to her what I was experiencing, although I omitted telling her that I had taken a short course of

Cipramil. I was still feeling quite ashamed yet I knew that Sue would not judge me.

'Okay. So let's talk about this a bit more,' she said, putting the kettle on and shredding a bunch of fresh herbs to make a pot of tea. 'Are you eating well?'

'Yes, like a horse, but I've lost pounds which I can't afford to lose,' I said, folding my arms to give me more bulk. She asked if I was drinking plenty of water and if my bowels were working. I nodded.

'And you've obviously been getting plenty of exercise. Too much, by the looks,' she said, eyeing my bag-of-bones body. 'Let's take our tea and go into my office. I want to do an iris diagnosis.' This showed low nervous energy, excess acidity and tired to very tired adrenals. (When the ovaries stop producing oestrogen, the adrenal glands become the main source of oestrogen production after menopause, albeit only producing a small amount. If the adrenals are under stress, this affects the tiny production of oestrogen.) She added these findings to the symptoms I had told her – insomnia, racing heart, tears, anxiety and feeling very fragile. She continued writing her notes while I sat sipping my interesting tea.

'I can see that you are physically and emotionally exhausted, Debra, and there are many combinations of herbs that I could use to help with that. But I'm also going to take into account your personality of being a perfectionist and an organiser,' she explained, and got up to prepare a bottle of what I call 'witch's brew'. In fact it was a herbal tonic and her prescription not only supported what was happening hormonally to me but it also helped to strengthened my resolve. In it were herbs of chamomile, alfalfa, vervain, yarrow, parsley, sage, hops and sarsaparilla.

Also Bach flowers of white chestnut, mustard, olive, beech, elm and red chestnut.

We sat a while longer and chatted in general terms about menopause. Sue is a great believer in getting rid of old negative stuff – recognise it, deal with it and chuck it away. 'Be positive and you will attract positivity and avoid illness,' she said as we parted.

Over the next couple of months I took my witch's brew, carefully measuring out the precise drops. It was revolting! A swig of port after the evening's dose made it more palatable. There was no miraculous effect, but I felt a little strength seeping through my veins. I ploughed through all the literature I had gathered, highlighting and making notes. I was astounded at the range of menopausal symptoms and also relieved that I could tick off many that I did not experience. But mine were listed in everything I read. The information also said that they are just some of the distressing symptoms that seventy-five per cent of women may encounter.

I am now in my mid fifties and it is five years since my symptoms first showed. I put on the lost kilos over three months and now maintain my normal weight. Fortunately, the herbal mixture works for me. I don't need it regularly. On the first occasion I took my drops twice a day for about five months until the bottle was empty. Then over three years lapsed before I felt that I needed to visit Sue again, my emotions fragile after another drop in oestrogen. This time round I knew what was happening to me. I could feel myself slipping and I visited the doctor and asked for a blood test which showed a measured drop in the hormone again. Sue's prescription was a little different this time, taking into account other events that were going on in my life, and I received immediate relief. It was far quicker than the first time round, perhaps because I had a greater understanding of myself and my belief in the herbs. I've never returned to antidepressants or needed to take HRT. This has not meant that I have 'renewed energy to fulfil ambitions and seize opportunities' as one brochure sees the beginning of this new phase in a woman's life. However, I am more my old self. My family can rely upon me in all things. There are rare times when I struggle with anxiety. It happens at night. I suddenly wake in the early hours of the morning in a panic, my heart racing, tears welling in my eyes, hot and sweaty. And I think to myself, 'Where the hell have you come from?' But I no longer fear it. I know it's part of the change that is still with me; for how much longer I do not know. Insomnia still troubles me. I can have a glorious day working in the garden, one of my joys, and be tired and ready to collapse. But it takes two hours to fall asleep, only to be woken at two and four in the morning, tossing and turning. I have developed a strategy which works fairly well for me. After a warm bath and a read in bed, I will allow myself half an hour to fidget, trying to turn off. And then I say to myself quite sternly, as if I'm a child, 'Right, now it's time to sleep.' And I concentrate on nothing but sleep. I refuse to allow my mind to wander anywhere else. It's not easy to do and it has taken me many months to master. My next discipline is to work on something that will keep me asleep, at least to string together five hours!

I have learnt to be open-minded on menopause. Every woman's menopause is different. I think a lot depends on what is going on in a woman's life at that time, the support she gets from family, friends and professionals, and her own personality and perception of herself. If I have a friend who uses HRT then I support her in her decision. And if another swears by wild yam cream, then I am glad for her too. As long as women are well informed then I believe their decision should be supported. I think, on balance, I have made the right decisions for me.

In managing my menopause I continue with my fitness routine at least twice a week which includes weight training, stretches, some aerobic and yoga classes. Work on the farm is hard, I dig holes and drag logs, plant and prune, all the while thinking, 'This is good for my bones.' I am very particular with my diet; everything is fresh, which means I shop daily for meat or fish, vegetables and fruit. I do not have a freezer, which drives my son mad. I rarely open a tin. I have a large herb garden and eat bunches of parsley and garlic cloves by the spoonful. I am mindful to keep my daily calcium intake high and include yoghurt, cheese, almonds and broccoli as well as high-calcium milk. My bone density is above average and I put this down to a lifetime of weight-bearing exercise and a variety of fresh food, and I thank my parents for good genes. I also have to give thanks to my friends. Their phone calls, lunches, walks, laughter and tears are treasured.

PENNY'S STORY

Mid-life can be a watershed in relationships, jobs and lifestyle. Menopause is part of all that. It certainly was part of Penny's menopause. The death of Penny's husband, the development of a new relationship, a change in job and the management of a new lifestyle all impacted on her menopause.

Menopause: n. the period of the cessation of menstruation. (*Macquarie Dictionary*)

This definition, as a means of describing the huge physical and emotional changes that took place in my life, is totally inadequate. Yet, before I embarked on my own voyage of menopause, I had no more understanding than that definition.

During all the years of my periods, I had the cyclical premenstrual tension where I changed from being placid Penny to the woman from hell. My family had to endure a miserable and moody week before the storm broke. My husband, John, and daughters wisely kept their distance from me and we all sighed with relief when my period arrived. Now we could enjoy life again – until next month!

During my forties, increased maturity and experience taught me to accept the waves of emotional and physical fluctuations as part of who I was. However, during this time, major life events were taking place around me. John's siblings were diagnosed with cancer: two died and one survived. My mother was diagnosed with Alzheimer's disease. When I was forty-three, John was diagnosed with his first melanoma. Seven years later he died from multiple metastatic melanoma.

Until John's death my monthly cycle continued in its own predictable way. But my sense of equilibrium quickly evaporated when he died. Within days I experienced my first hot flush. I recognised it for what is was – my first meeting with menopause. I kicked the blankets off, only to pull them up again, cold and shivering. Also my periods did not arrive on their due date. 'Great! Not only have I got learn to live without John, even my bloody periods have gone,' I thought. My periods had been a source of reassurance that at least my body was staying the same when everything else around me had changed. Now my regular, reliable body rhythms had let me down. Six weeks after John's death, my period made a brief visit. I was sitting, sobbing on the bathroom floor when I noticed the spotting. This time I was angry because they had come back! The next day I saw my doctor who assured me that my body was physically responding to the grief.

Over the following months, my periods gradually returned to their monthly rhythm and I soon learned to predict when it was crying time. Any grief I had been trying to control in the previous three weeks, flooded over me in a tidal wave when my hormone levels dropped. I cried all day. It was a relief to let it all go. By the end of the first year of widowhood, I was learning to deal with living on my own and I started to meet new people. My periods were regular again and my mood swings had subsided.

However, I was uncertain about my future and had times of high anxiety and low confidence that often made me feel emotionally fragile. I believe I was experiencing a combination of hormonal changes and real-life changes. The difference between the two is sometimes indistinguishable.

About two years after John died, I met Kevin. Kevin fully understood my pain and grief—and I his. We had both lost a spouse. We were able to express and share our feelings of sadness and felt completely comfortable with each other. A beautiful relationship was developing. I visited my doctor again and, although the chances of pregnancy were small, we agreed that I would take oral contraceptives. The pill not only gave me protection it also stabilised my emotions. It helped me to make sensible decisions on my future, especially with a new relationship.

While I took the pill, menopause 'paused'. Six months later a gynaecologist advised me to cease taking the pill and allow my body to show where it was on its menopausal journey. Six weeks later I had a ten-day period. That was it, over. I waited each month but they never returned. To my surprise I felt no sadness—more relief. I accepted that this part of my life cycle had come, given me children and had now departed.

Other symptoms of menopause returned, hot flushes and disrupted sleep. I could fall asleep, but then woke for a loo visit and lay thinking about small issues, past and current, until they became mountains. Anxiety would arrive and settle in. Frustrated, I would get out of bed, make a cup of chamomile tea, and play computer games until I felt calmer. I would return to bed, fall into a deep sleep, only to be jolted by the shrill of the alarm clock. I woke, daunted with the prospect of having to deal with another day. Ten minutes of meditation, a pep talk to myself, showering and dressing were basic but necessary steps to overcome my anxiety. Although I feared the daily challenge ahead of me, I carried on in my profession as a registered nurse. Patients' needs gave me little time to think about myself.

Weekends were the hardest. I needed the distraction of social events, family and friends. The anxiety attacks tortured me night after night until I told myself to 'Stop!' Sometimes I succeeded in letting go; other times the anxiety gnawed at me like a rat. The constant anxiety attacks, hot flushes and broken sleep soon had me feeling out of control as I struggled to deal with changes resulting from John's death. I was grieving and angry, aware that he was at times a convenient target for my difficulty in dealing with life issues, which may have occurred anyway. On the other hand, feeling out of control could also have been a release valve for unexpressed grief. I felt the pressure from society to be 'over it' after a year had passed, and to resume a normal life (whatever that is). Kevin was a godsend with his patience and good humour. He understood that grief would resurface again and again over the years – a sick daughter, a child's twenty-first birthday, a major decision that would have been shared as a family. He knew, too, that such events would take me back to the beginning, with tears and sadness, but that with each occurrence the recovery time would be a little faster.

Tired of struggling against these turbulent emotions, I began to seek out ways of coping more effectively. To my surprise I discovered that hydration played a significant part in managing my anxiety. I started to drink a glass of water every hour. Several trips to the loo later and more glasses of water, I could feel my anxiety lift and a sense of exhaustion and almost euphoria set in. Perhaps I was flushing out toxins that were affecting my emotions. Walking also helped. It was more effective if I walked with a friend as it distracted me from any negative thoughts. Alone, I walked and worried at the same time. I was absorbed in self-pity until I could take no more. I told myself, 'Stop! Get over it! Appreciate your loving family and supportive friends, your good health and a beautiful world. Cut it out!' While I remained vigilant to this routine, my symptoms were less intrusive on my everyday life.

Kevin and I decided to fulfil our dream of a five-month trip around Australia in a caravan. He was a brave man travelling with a menopausal woman – moody, emotional and bitchy. At the end of a long day and several hundreds of kilometres, I was impatient, irritable and unreasonable. I often surprised myself at how snappy I could be. It was unlike me, unfamiliar ground. Here I was, in a new relationship, and exploring all my emotions, unrestrained! Kevin's patience and support never failed and this gave me the security to test the boundaries.

One afternoon, driving towards Darwin, we followed a recommendation to stay at Daly Waters Hotel, an outback place with 'plenty of character' that had a camping facility. I was not keen. I visualised a dusty dump, drunks, filth and flies. After refuelling at Elliot, an hour before the turnoff for Daly Waters, we drove past a modern motel. I looked longingly, but Kevin drove on. I sulked. We arrived at Daly Waters late in the day when most camping spots were occupied. Kevin was considerate, parking the caravan near the facilities for my convenience. 'We have to move,' I snapped. 'It stinks.' He moved our rig. After setting up,

Kevin told me that he had left the petrol cap back in Elliot. I exploded. Kevin walked away to the pub, returning a few minutes later with a petrol cap in hand. Still livid, and now ashamed of my behaviour, I said nothing and stormed off to the toilets. Returning, I tripped and fell on my face, and cried like a child. I picked myself up and went back to Kevin who looked puzzled at this child-woman wailing in front of him. Later, calm and with a glass of wine, I asked Kevin how he had found a petrol cap that fitted. The 'wonderful Daly Waters' had a cardboard box full of such treasures needing a home for people like us.

When Kevin and I returned from our trip I recognised that I needed advice and treatment to help me through menopause. Hormone replacement was not an option as my mother's twin sister had died from breast cancer. I made an appointment to see a naturopath. She showed me how to nurture myself and counselled me to meet the physical needs of my body. She helped me to build my confidence, to make choices that suited me, and to accept change. Treatment was healing-based through empowerment. I had a lot to learn and success came gradually. I rewrote the rules and, for the first time in my life, started to do things my way. I could say, 'No thanks, I do not want to do that.' I did not allow others to pressure me and I no longer feared disapproval. The naturopath taught me to look at menopause as a process, a passage of one part of my life to another. I began to focus less on the symptoms and when I suffered a bout of anxiety I accepted it as part of my being. Although the naturopath did not prescribe any medication (natural or otherwise) I took evening primrose oil capsules and tried several natural supplements for menopause. The only one that worked was Promensil. It was so effective that I thought I was through menopause and stopped taking it. I was wrong. Hot flushes returned and anxiety rose.

Later in menopause my libido started to fluctuate. However, I refuse to get hung up over this. I am in a loving relationship with Kevin and we are both philosophical about my changes. We enjoy intimacy and I know how to show him that he is loved. The bottle of lubricant sits in the bedside drawer to help with dryness. My face is now looking a little more lived-in these days, but I do not fret about this either. I have facials, drink lots of water and I smile. Kevin loves my smile, wrinkles and all. During my menopausal years my weight increased. Was it the wine and seafood platters? Was it hormonal? At first I avoided looking at myself in mirrors and wore loose-fitting clothes but now I am taking responsibility to slim down a few kilos.

I am nearly at the end of my menopause and it has been a rite of passage. Sometimes I still wake with anxiety but often relate this to mental overload. I pull myself back into line and tell myself that I cannot be superwoman. I work hard at keeping a balance between work, relationships, leisure and time for myself. When the balance is not right, physical and mental symptoms will manifest themselves. I am stronger at managing the challenges in my life and as my confidence and security increase, the time to process these changes decreases. The understanding and insight I have gained through this menopausal maze has more than compensated for the emotional and physical discomfort that accompanied it. I am more at peace with myself than I have ever been, more complete. I feel blessed.

Penny is now in her mid to late fifties. She manages an allied-health day therapy centre that services a retirement village and the wider community. In addition to Promensil, she takes calcium and magnesium, and has mammograms and bone density scans. Penny is grateful for Kevin's support, and his patience, during her menopause. Her daughters tell her she is spoilt.

PEARL'S STORY

As well as managing the audit for an on-farm food safety program and administering her partner's manufacturing business, Pearl has worked in senior sales and marketing roles. Recently she acknowledged that she could no longer handle the high pressure as well as menopause. Pearl, now fifty-three, has spent the last thirteen years battling menopause. It has impacted on her life in many ways.

What I miss most as I go through menopause is feeling joy. Sometimes it makes a fleeting appearance but I miss waking in the morning and really looking forward to the day. I want to swing my legs out from the bed, stretch myself tall and throw my wardrobe door open to plan what to wear. I want to smile in the mirror and say, you look good today, slip on a pair of high heels and rush out the door feeling carefree.

Instead, I'm exhausted before the day has begun. I've had another sleepless night and my body is aching. I make some coffee and push open the kitchen window. It's seven in the morning and the mist rolls and swirls among the vines. I welcome the earthy fresh air into the kitchen and give a little shudder of pleasure. I want this feeling to last all day, but moments later I'm feeling flat. Joy. Where did joy go? Today, I don't have to get ready for work; it's my flexi-day and Anna is coming around for lunch and a chat. I pick up a little at the thought. Anna and I met some twenty years ago when we were awarded a free holiday in Sydney. Since then we have been solid friends, catching up regularly over a meal, often with other girlfriends. I can always rely on these meetings for uninhibited laughter and gossip. Anna is two years older than me and our menopauses have overlapped, each of us experiencing similar symptoms.

I was perimenopausal when I was about forty. I don't know why I was so early, but my periods became erratic, occurring any time between fifteen and thirty-one days, and I started to have very heavy periods with flooding. I also started to have hot flushes and night sweats, although at forty they were not regular. Two years later I became aware of escalating depression which I relate to the increasing menopausal symptoms. I put up with the frustration and inconvenience until I was about forty-eight when I saw a female gynaecologist who prescribed Provera. I have suffered from severe migraines since I was sixteen and whilst on Provera the headaches increased to fourteen days per month and the pain was unbearable. I also had spotting nearly every day with Provera which was intolerable. I stopped taking it after three months.

I can hear that George is up. I walk to the back door and can see that the fluorescent lights are on in the shed. I put a croissant into the microwave for him and pour steaming black coffee into a mug. I leave my slippers by the door and put my feet into wellies and take a tray out. I notice that it has rained over night. George has his head down the belly of an old Fergusson tractor that he is restoring. He's brilliant at this sort of thing; if you can't buy it he'll make it, and if it's broken he'll fix it. But he's not good on the listening front, or talking about personal matters. I suppose it's a male thing but I do wish he would put his arm around me and say, 'How are you going?' I think he just assumes that I'm travelling along okay, or is it that he doesn't really care? Do men want to understand? I don't know of many women who have been able to pour their heart out to their partner and get sympathetic understanding and help with their menopause. Perhaps it's my fault. I have always been organised in business and on the home front, and if anything is worrying or upsetting me I suppress my emotions. I've been burying negative feelings since childhood and I've continued to do this in my relationship. But George knows I'm not okay. I say good morning and a hand appears to acknowledge that I have left a tray. I walk back to the house, feeling heavy. Not one word!

I didn't receive much understanding or sympathy from the specialist who prescribed Provera either, so I changed and saw a male gynaecologist who performed a curette when I was forty-nine and suggested I try a Mirena IUD, a form of birth control designed to help people who bleed heavily. It works by delivering small doses of hormones direct to the uterus and lasts for five years. The gynaecologist told me that the Mirena IUD would stop my bleeding completely. Although it did stop the flooding, I continued to have light periods with some break-through bleeding. The periods fluctuated from fifteen to sixty-four days in the first three years and now, in the fourth year, I feel my periods are definitely coming to an end. I can tell when a period is coming because I get sore breasts and a headache. Apart from that, the Mirena has been fantastic. I have one more year to go before the IUD is taken out and the specialist expects me to be through menopause by then. I will be fifty-five and I hope he is right!

I plan to make a banana cake for after lunch. From the fridge door I grab the milk, nestled up next to the Windex. I have been searching for that everywhere. I see the funny side and then I frown. Recently I forgot to eat my usual breakfast before leaving for work. Another day I couldn't find my handbag. I worried and searched all day at work wondering where I had left it. When I got home it was on the kitchen table. I was so relieved, but what's happening to me?

When I turned fifty-one I had been experiencing menopause on and off for about thirteen years. I had light infrequent periods, thanks to the IUD, but I was increasingly suffering from a number of symptoms: anxiety, depression, confusion and forgetfulness, tiredness and body pain. My GP received the results of blood tests and diagnosed menopause. He made no suggestions about what I could do or what I could take. No doctor I have seen has pushed HRT, which has surprised me, as other friends have experienced the opposite. He used a lot of medical terms about the physiological aspects of menopause but nothing about how menopause could affect me emotionally, although he indicated that my anxiety could be related to menopause.

The feelings of loss and sadness from this news came later. I cried alone. No more the young girl feeling like I have my whole life ahead of me. I thought of attractive girls and boys enjoying their excited youth, all those highs around romance and sexuality. Will there be romance again with George? Immediately after that news, I had five twenty-eight-day cycles with normal periods. So much for the blood test results.

The kitchen is warm and has a wonderful aroma of sweet baking. I busy myself with planning the lunch. A range of cheeses, I think, and a jar of my own spicy chutney and homemade quince jelly. I write a note to buy leg ham and a crusty loaf. The dishes are quickly washed and the benches wiped of speckled flour. The sav blanc! I forgot to put it in the fridge last night. Damn. A quick look at the clock says nearly ten. Already!

I feel anxiety rise from the pit of my stomach. I try to calm down, reminding myself that it's only Anna coming for lunch, and she *will* understand. My anxiety levels have increased immensely in the last couple of years. Feelings of not coping bring on my anxiety. It is mostly work related, although I am currently going through a patch where I can't seem to get through the housework and shopping. I like to be on top of things, organised and prepared. I hate people just dropping in, yet I usually enjoy their company. It's a love/hate thing. When they leave, I look around and see all the unfinished jobs and my anxiety rises.

I grab my purse and let the door slam behind me. As I'm getting into the car I shout to George that I'm off to the shops. Halfway there I realise I have forgotten to pick up my note. What was it I had to buy? What am I doing for lunch? I keep driving, racking my brain. I'm definitely not thinking clearly. Sometimes these situations are funny and I can laugh at them, but they are also a source of worry. Anna and I both suffer from anxiety, but we're different. I perspire when anxious, she doesn't. She has heart palpitations and sometimes her chest feels tight and it slightly hurts. It's only when I see the bakery that I remember a crusty loaf and ham. I try to think of anything else that I was supposed to get; did George ask me to get him something? I wait in the queue to pay, conscious of the time ticking by, feeling panic rising.

When I get home I fly through the door and finish preparing lunch. Half an hour to go. I shower and apply my makeup carefully and dress for a casual Sunday lunch. I hear Anna's car on the gravel and she gets out carrying a bottle of wine. The sav blanc! It's still in the wine rack. Shit!

'Anna! Hi, come in,' I say and thank her for the wine, a red. Oh well! She plonks her bag, sunnies and keys on the sideboard and says that the drive to Margaret River was beautiful. 'I'd love to have a walk around the place, Pearl. Are you up to it?' she asks, knowing of my body pain.

My body pain started slowly with the onset of menopause at forty but has increased markedly since I turned fifty-two. I am pleased to say that my body only gives me as much pain as I can bear. It's either my upper body – hands, wrists, elbows, shoulders and neck – or my lower body – ribs, hips, thighs, legs and feet. Pain is usually a constant dull ache, but it can be sharp like a toothache. It lasts for a couple of months with no relief and the brief spells of no pain are diminishing. I am stiff, despite doing a lot of stretching and flexibility exercises with yoga. I don't sleep well, some nights not at all, and I believe this and the accompanying tiredness contribute to my body pain. As does anxiety, especially when I tense up. And I have pain from arthritis in my knees and hips, and I worry about what my life will be like in the future.

Anna and I walk down a slight hill and open a gate, mindful to close it behind us so that the cattle don't wander through the vines. Tiny green grapes are hanging in bunches waiting for warm sunny days to ripen them. Anna asks me how my migraines are and I tell her that they are becoming less frequent and less severe. Anna, too, has been a long-time sufferer of migraines and we agree that all the different migraine medications and giving up the trigger foods did not help, but that a change in hormones has. It's about the only positive thing to menopause.

We climb a hill and exchange other news: the ding to the back of her car, courtesy of her daughter; her son's failure in three of four subjects at second year uni.

'I'm not sure what's harder, Pearl, a teenage daughter with enough emotions and tears and tantrums to fuel a nuclear plant, or a son whose main focus (if he knows what the word means) is sleep and computer games. Nicky never stops talking and I can't get a word from Hugh. I really do wonder how they can be so different.' When we reach a bit of flat land and get our breath back we have a good laugh. Laughing is not easy these days for me. I still laugh with people, but not on my own. If I watch a comedy on TV on my own I don't laugh, but if I am with George I do. It's a strange thing, but when I do laugh it is such a release.

George and I made the decision not to have children. We have been involved in our respective careers and the decision has never bothered us. When I hear friends anguish over their kids I think some women get a double or triple whammy. Menopause and kids and partner!

'By the way, I took your advice about using Vagifem,' Anna says. 'I asked the doctor if there were any risks with long-term use and she said that she has women in their eighties and nineties using them. I must have given her an incredulous look because she laughed and said, not for intercourse, just for relief!'

I lost my libido at a younger age than most and I don't know why. I was about thirty-seven. I experienced an extremely dry vagina and bouts of cystitis. Even using tampons became difficult. Although it was an issue then, George's libido is (fortunately) at the same level as mine now. I use vaginal pessaries that release a little oestrogen and they make a difference. I have experienced problems with incontinence since then too. A physiotherapist who specialises in incontinence taught me how to do pelvic floor exercises properly and I do these faithfully at least three times a day. I have also cut down on the amount of fluid I drink each day. I was drinking eight glasses of water and about the same in tea and coffee, and the physio thought this was too much for my body.

'Did you try Melatonin?' I ask Anna. We have both had chronic sleeping problems, lying awake for hours, or suddenly jolting awake after only two hours' sleep. I have tried prescribed medication and slept well the first night but subsequent nights I still woke every hour. It also left me groggy during the day.

'Yes, but I don't always sleep. It relaxes me and I guess I have to be grateful for that,' Anna says and I agree with her.

'Of course the night sweats don't help and I think my body is getting used to Menohealth, just like it got used to Femular, although both worked well at the start,' says Anna who seems to be having a hot flush just talking about them.

Anna asks me how my part-time job is going. My aim is to reduce my working hours in an attempt to reduce stress and to have some time to myself although I have yet to find the time to laze around, put my feet up and read.

I am currently working part-time in aged care, the duties are varied and I need the people contact. Still, sometimes I don't feel that I am functioning properly and I get over-whelmed.

'Perhaps you should think about retiring, Pearl?' Anna suggests, after I tell her of my recent outburst to management.

'No, I think that if I were at home I would fall further down the hole of depression. I need routine and I need people contact, even if they do anger me sometimes. I don't know where to go next for help with depression. I've stopped taking antidepressants. None worked for me. Did I tell you that I became jittery and my feet started to tap when I was taking them? I slept even less and stopped feeling.'

'What do you mean, "You stopped feeling"?' Anna asks, full of concern.

'Well, I rarely cry these days. I've suppressed my emotions for so long that my tears seemed to have dried up.'

'Wish I could say the same,' Anna says. 'I cry bucket-loads, heaving and sobbing until I can barely open my eyes. Sometimes, the tears just seep all day long like a leaking tap. I'm so glad I can talk to you about these things, Pearl. I'm still very careful whom I tell because a lot of people look on depression as a weakness or a mental problem. It's not just me or you; it's a whole lot of people out there.'

We are walking back along a worn track made by the cattle, passing hundreds of gums that George and I planted many years ago. Anna loops her arm through mine and we are quiet for a while. I'm feeling more relaxed in my friend's company, feeling hungry and looking forward to a glass of wine. Bugger the white! We reach the shed and pop our heads around the door to tell George that lunch will be in twenty minutes. He looks up and nods, wiping his hands on a greasy rag.

'How is George?' Anna asks when we enter the kitchen. It's a loaded question. She knows it and I know it.

'Actually, I had a bit of a breakdown recently,' I tell Anna and she puts an arm around me. 'George was quite shocked. I felt like asking him, "Do I need to have a breakdown to get any reaction from you?" I know I tend to keep things to myself, but I have mentioned to him what I am going through and it's as if he hasn't heard me. He doesn't know how to comfort me, Anna. When I had a week off on stress leave, and saw a counsellor, he never asked once how it was all going.'

Anna listens attentively. She says that she understands and I know that she does. Not only because of the menopause but she, too, has a husband who is unable or unwilling to try and understand.

It seems to me that even if a woman is difficult, negative and sad, her friendships with other women will remain strong. Yet her relationship with her partner can suffer. Perhaps it's because men don't have menopause and therefore cannot truly understand. Perhaps it's because they are trying to cope with their own mid-life issues.

Anna and I put the plates on the table and I ask her what she'd like to drink.

'Oh, I think a cold glass of white would go down very well with the lovely spread you've prepared,' she says.

'Well, the only cold I've got is Windex!' I say, taking it out of the fridge door and holding it up. I tell her the story and she roars with laughter.

'Do you remember your last trip to BreastScreen?' she splutters, 'When you wore one black shoe and one navy shoe.' We are both holding our stomachs laughing loudly when George walks in. He grabs the bottle of red and uncorks it, all the while bewildered with our hysteria. But I can see that he's pleased to see two happy women – for a change!

It is still an up and down road for Pearl. Her weekly exercise routine of yoga, walking and light weights assist in the management of her menopause. She has regular physiotherapy, remedial massage and occasional chiropractic treatment but is still searching for a solution to her body pain. Counselling helps with depression that she associates with menopause and the loss of youth.

Her recent breakdown shocked George and he's showing great consideration. He helps in the kitchen, books a restaurant and takes time out for a Sunday drive. He recognises that their property is a lot of work and that it was his dream, not Pearl's, and has offered to give it up for a more manageable place. Best of all, he now asks, 'How are you today?'

TO MY FIFTIES

There was a time I'd have snubbed you in the street,
skittered past like a snippet of conversation.
Then when you had me in your sights like a hurtling truck,
your traytop rattling about on rusting rivets,
I hoped you'd never make it round the last bend.
But now that you're here and you've unpacked
your censorious sighs and thinning hair,
now that you've given truth to the rumour of gravitational
    gravitas,
(and flesh to the humour of a belly laugh)
I find I don't mind you at all.
With you menopaused beside me, I can call a spade
a bloody shovel and blame it on the mad woman
in the attic. I can flirt with the boy behind the counter
at the coffee shop and know for certain (and with the
    utmost relief)
he won't be asking for my number.
I can count my blessings and know that good health,
two children reared safely into their twenties,
and not living in a war zone,
equals an abundance indeed.
So settle down, my dear fifties.
Put your head on my shoulder and rest a while.

Yes, I know the sixties aren't far away
but most of them still have their eye on the future,
their children have left home (for now at least),
and I've seen their super payouts and retirement plans.
Take it from me – they're a push over!

Louise Nicholas

GAYE'S STORY

Gaye's menopausal experiences have been extraordinary. Her journey starts when she was a teenager and as a consequence of her health issues, her menopause began at thirty-two.

I was sixteen when I was diagnosed with Hodgkin's disease (cancer of the lymphatic system), and treated with radio-therapy. I went into remission – a reprieve of the disease that could last months, years and hopefully forever. In my youthful naivety I thought I was invincible anyway, that the doctors were all wrong and the tests were somehow wrong, too. I'd even been excited about being admitted into the ward: free accommodation and room service! I went shopping with Mum for a brightly coloured dressing gown in honour of the event and saw it as a holiday from my long hours as a hairdressing apprentice. When I finally left hospital some nine months and several operations later I had a different view of my vacation. For the next five years I got on with my life and at twenty-one I began to feel unwell as the symptoms of the disease began to recur. The remission was over. I was back fighting for my life. I began a gruelling six-month course of chemotherapy which turned out to be a complete cure for the disease. I had a second chance at life.

I met my partner shortly after and I was twenty-three when we bought a house and started to think about having children. My periods were irregular and painful and when three years passed with no pregnancy, I was sent for tests. One ovary had been removed many years earlier because of a cyst and the results showed that the fallopian tube, leading to my one remaining ovary, was blocked. We were referred to the IVF program and at twenty-seven I was placed on a long waiting list. Another two years passed during which time I had a test which showed that my remaining ovary had a cyst and my uterus had a fibroid but the doctors assured me that I would be alright and my turn would come soon enough.

I had been state manager for a credit card company and enjoyed the responsibility although the days were long and travel was regular. The job demanded me to be alert, focused and energetic but around this time I began having trouble sleeping. At night I was restless, tossing and turning with an uncontrollable urge to wriggle and move my legs. I felt crawling sensations under my skin and, burning hot, I'd kick off all the blankets, turn on the air conditioner and literally freeze my skin so that I could cool down enough to get some sleep. I was so tired that the days were a struggle. But I forced myself to run on empty.

I was feeling pressure from my job and pressure waiting for IVF and worrying that my ovary would be eaten away before I got the chance to use my eggs. I put my insomnia and night sweats down to these stresses. In addition, I had not had a period for six months and I suspected something was wrong. I made an appointment to see my doctor, fretting and thinking, 'What now?' After a simple blood test I was told the grim news that I was clinically menopausal, at the age of thirty-two. I learned that premature menopause can be a consequence of radiotherapy. Even though I still had my uterus, my surviving ovary had shut down and ceased to produce oestrogen. No oestrogen! What about my eggs? What about my baby? Wasn't that the very hormone that made me a woman? How on earth could I get by without it? What was going to happen to me? I went through emotional anguish: panic, anger and a huge sense of loss. Why me? Was I going to age and become a granny overnight? What would happen to my hair, my skin, my body? I felt as though I had been robbed of my youth. Wasn't menopause a thing that happened to women who had finished their child-bearing years? They were fifty, weren't they? I had never been warned that this could happen to me and I admit feeling very sorry for myself.

My doctor immediately started me on hormone replacement therapy – very high doses of oestrogen pills and also progesterone vaginal pessaries. This regime was necessary in order to emulate the hormones that I had produced premenopause. I had an immediate response to the treatment. I felt normal, my old self. Wonderfully sane again. But my happiness was short-lived. I had to be placed on a different IVF waiting list as I now needed donor eggs; I received no credit for the years waiting on the previous IVF program.

Finally, after eight long years of early morning appointments for injections and blood tests, seven failed IVF attempts and a myriad of tests, I conceived a beautiful boy, followed two years later by a precious baby girl. After the children were born the dosage of my HRT was reduced. The high levels of oestrogen were no longer necessary.

When my daughter was about eight months old I had to have a radical hysterectomy to remove my uterus – due to endometriosis, a painful condition of the lining – and my remaining ovary. I was sent home without HRT and after a few days the symptoms of the menopause returned with a vengeance. I had terrible insomnia, night after night. I felt depressed, tired, exhausted and afraid. I telephoned my doctor after a few weeks of hell and was told, 'Oops! Forgot to put you back on Premarin.' I started again on the oestrogen and the awful feelings lessened considerably – enough to bring my life back to normal and to concentrate on being a good mum again.

My partner and I owned five bakeries and I left my position with the credit card company to manage the book-keeping aspects of the business. Sometimes I also helped out in the shops during late-night trading and on weekends, or if a staff member was sick. It was a seven days a week job. Life was extremely hectic. Although I was on HRT, the symptoms of menopause did not leave me entirely. I still had the occasional sweaty, sleepless night, I was losing a worrying amount of hair and my skin was noticeably drier. I felt that the symptoms of menopause were exacerbated by the stresses of my daily life. At times I was unclear whether the cause was menopause or stress. Menopause was some-thing that I could not share with my girlfriends. I had to handle this without them, trusting in my doctors. I was not even forty years old and I was trying to juggle a young family, run a business with my partner, and cope with my health issues, including menopause. I was not prepared for the shattering events which followed.

My father was diagnosed with multiple myeloma. He had been a handsome and fit man of sixty-four when the six months of chemotherapy turned him into an emaciated old man. It was hoped that the treatment would give him five years. There was a new treatment, in its experimental stage, which the doctors thought might give him a longer, if not indefinite, remission. He was considered to be a prime candidate and encouraged to try. Who wouldn't grasp at the opportunity of life?

Unfortunately, the treatment went horribly wrong and damaged his kidneys and liver. Despite being sorry, the doctors said that there was nothing they could do except place him on life support. My proud and intelligent father refused and wanted to return home and die with dignity. I nursed him for those two last days, administering his pain-killing injections and praying that he wasn't suffering. Standing beside his bed, my gently sobbing mother, my grief-stricken brothers and I watched him pass away.

This loss was closely followed by the news that my partner had been having an affair with one of my brother's wives. Both marriages ended abruptly. My children were four and two years old. I was missing my dear father and had to cope with my ex-partner's aggressive and threatening behaviour because I would not consider a reconciliation. The next two years were very difficult. I moved three times into rental properties until finally returning to the family home after a marital settlement. It was unsettling for my children going from the security and tradition of two parents living together, to a sharing arrangement. I started a new period of soul searching and tried my best to give my children the best I could. Beginning a single life again at forty was a profoundly difficult thing for me. I was forty and menopausal! I found the whole situation alarming and uncomfortable and sometimes crazy. I knew that life was meant to be shared and that I was not meant to be alone forever.

As I neared forty-two I was advised to cut back on my oestrogen which was considered to be at dangerously high levels. Long-term use of oestrogen replacement therapy had been associated with an increased risk of breast cancer and I was already at high risk because of the radiotherapy treatment in my teens. There is also an increased risk of blood clotting and strokes. I still had small residual patches of endometriosis after my hysterectomy and these patches acted adversely in the presence of high levels of oestrogen. However, the use of HRT was recommended in an attempt to reduce the risk of osteoporosis and heart disease. As the levels of oestrogen decreased, so the symptoms reappeared – not as severely as when I had no oestrogen but nevertheless they were distressing.

At the age of forty-six I met a man. My sexual relationship with him caused a vicious cycle of urinary tract infections treated by antibiotics which caused thrush. My vagina was dry. Orgasm was difficult. And having sex in the first place is impossible when you are treating yourself for thrush or if you have cystitis. My doctor told me that I had a general thinning and atrophy of my genital/urinary tissues due to the loss of oestrogen and this was causing the dryness and the recurrent UTIs. These frequent infections made me depressed and anxious about my new relationship. That in itself was a deterrent in the bedroom. The effects of early menopause made me self-conscious about the way I looked and my confidence was low. How could I have a normal relationship when I had something wrong with me all the time? I was always apologising for being unable to make love.

I was referred to an urologist who told me nothing that I hadn't already discovered during my many hours of scouring the internet. Pee after sex, not before. Wash after sex. Drink cranberry juice. Try half an antibiotic tablet within an hour or so of sex. Use low dose oestrogen pessaries twice a week to help the vaginal tissues make their own natural lubricant and make penetration easier. Can you imagine the scene? 'Oh, hang on, I've just got to take a pill with a glass of cranberry juice.' And instead of lying in my lover's arms warm in the afterglow of unbridled passionate love, I must jump up and run to the loo to wash all the evidence away immediately only to return to bed to find him snoring! How romantic! The prophylactic antibiotic gave me thrush anyway and so the cycle repeated itself. The relationship ended, but not solely because of the problems in the bedroom. He found a younger woman. I put that down to menopause, too!

I looked older than my forty-seven years. My skin was dry and prematurely wrinkled. My once luxuriously thick hair had been shedding heavily for a few years and looked thin and frizzy. My hairdressers prescribed expensive conditioners and treatments but to no avail. I tried vitamins and various supplements. You name them, I tried them, but the hair loss continued and still does to this day.

And I was single again. I wondered how I could contemplate a relationship if I couldn't make love with my partner? What man would want a celibate relationship? I searched for information on menopause and especially the urinary tract infections that were, in my experience, one of the most debilitating side effects of menopause. I read about a cream called Estriol that could be used vaginally instead of pessaries. It contained a different type of oestrogen. I asked my doctor for a prescription. Curiously, at no time had any doctor suggested this cream as a potential remedy for my condition; a condition that was consuming my life, reaping havoc with my body and causing me immense distress. Miraculously my infections stopped. I was elated.

Alleviating dryness is vital to avoid urinary tract infections and to help with comfortable intercourse. I also think that a caring, gentle approach to lovemaking when you are menopausal makes for a less problematic physical response. For me, menopause has been an on-going exercise in gleaning information from every possible source. I found doctors reluctant to discuss or take seriously any of the side effects of menopause such as dry skin, hair loss and loss of muscle and skin tone. I was made to feel that these changes are considered as vanity and something that I should not be complaining about. These 'put downs' only made me more anxious and self conscious; they are certainly unhelpful.

I continue to take Premarin tablets, however hot flushes are still with me in the evenings. I am currently trialling evening primrose oil as a remedy for my dry skin and hair and also for relief from the flushes, although I have not had much success to date. But it's early days. My skin is sometimes so hot at night that the wonderful new love of my life of two years cannot touch me and is astounded by the amount of heat radiating from my body. I have found that magnesium supplements help to prevent the cramps that sometimes have me jumping from the bed in the middle of the night, scaring the pants off my loving partner. Calcium supplements reduce my risk of osteoporosis, a condition that I am at high risk of because of the radiotherapy and early menopause. Vitamin C helps to reduce the easy bruising and occasionally bursting blood vessels in my fingers which I have read is caused by the thinning of the blood vessel walls and the general decline in the efficiency of the circulatory system as a result of menopause. Vitamin B12 and the rest of the B group vitamins improve the quality of my hair. Zinc is also deficient after menopause and an important factor in hair growth as well as boosting the immune system and increasing resistance to infections. My medicine cabinet is bursting with vitamins, pills and potions. In addition to the supplements I take, exercise is a vital part of my regime. To protect my bone density I do weight-bearing exercises and use hand weights, barbells and dumbbells. Walking is another. My bi-annual mammogram is a necessary intrusion and one that I never miss, although I dislike it intensely. There is something undignified – not to mention painful – about squashing your breasts flat between two panes of glass and stretching your skin until you think it's going to rip apart – but I am at high risk and never miss an appointment. I shall not complain! Bone density examinations are another bi-annual event.

As much as I feel sorry for myself from time to time I count my blessings, especially my two children who were a miracle and a gift. And now that I approach fifty and my friends begin to feel the effects of menopause I'm able to empathise and offer worthy advice, from experience. If only I could drag a bit of fat from my hips and implant it in my boobs! My menopausal friends and I can laugh about our saggy bits and under-the-cover tricks.

I also feel blessed in sharing my life with a supportive and loving man who understands and accepts that I am not in my twenties, trim, taut and terrific, and just bursting with oestrogen. I am nearly fifty, menopausal, and my life is a whole lot better than it was before.

For the past two years Gaye has been an administrator for a large childcare centre. She recently sold her house with all the memories of her past, and she has bought another with promises of a fresh start. After many years Gaye is contented, secure in a relationship and looking forward to a brighter future.

JENNY'S STORY

Jenny is post-menopause and in her mid to late fifties. She and Martin have been married for over thirty years and they have no children. For most of her working life Jenny was employed in the Melbourne state office of a federal government department. Her menopause started at thirty-nine. It may have been hereditary but Jenny wonders if shock played a part in her early menopause.

'If I'm like my mother during menopause, you can shoot me,' I'd say to my husband in my twenties and thirties when a bad dose of PMT gave me a foretaste of what I thought menopausal mood swings would be like. Mum's menopause was pretty gruelling for her and for our family. She had terrible fits of depression when, for days or weeks at a time, she would sit in her bedroom apparently unable to bring herself to do anything around the house or talk to her family. When she did get herself together and go out, she would often be caught short at the shops or in some other public place by an unexpected menstrual flood. The unreliable periods ended when, at the age of forty-five, she had a hysterectomy, the popular solution to menopausal difficulties in the early 1970s, although the moodiness continued for many years.

After my mother's experience I wasn't looking forward to menopause. In the event, it came upon me quite gently, if at a much younger age than I expected. I was thirty-nine. It may have been hereditary as my mother and grand-mother both went through the change of life in their early to mid forties, or it may have been shock induced. My cycle changed after our house and garden were devastated by a flash flood that was as unexpected as it was shocking given that we live on a hill, not a riverbank. Drains blocked by hail channelled a huge wall of water overland which knocked down our back fence, ripped the side off the garage and spread muck throughout the garden and house. It took months to clean up the debris and to repair the damage.

My periods had always been regular and uneventful, but after the flood I started to experience occasional irregularity. This irregularity became the norm from the age of forty-two to forty-six. I was never sure when my period would come next – a week or six weeks later. At one time I had three periods in five weeks and although I felt sure it was menopause, I visited the doctor because I was worried that I had some terrible bleeding illness. However, I was assured that it was menopause.

I had a three-month run of hot flushes when I was forty-four, then a whole year's worth before my periods finally stopped when I was forty-six. I thought I had escaped menopause pretty lightly. Manageable periods and no mood swings. The hot flushes had been inconvenient and occasionally embarrassing but they hadn't bothered me much. A few bouts of night sweats or too many periods close together would leave me light-headed. But generally I had felt pretty good – fit, healthy and optimistic.

After my last period, I made an appointment with my doctor for a checkup and to discuss a delicate matter. Intercourse had become raspy and painful for me, an ordeal. Although I could discuss this with Martin, my husband, I worried about how it might affect our relationship. I sat in the doctor's room, feeling quite embarrassed as I explained my symptoms. My doctor was a man in his sixties and I didn't expect his response.

'It's time for you to take HRT,' he said. 'My wife's on HRT and she likes it. I like it! She's a bit of a tigress in bed,' he confided with relish.

I hadn't realised that a dry vagina and painful intercourse were common problems for menopausal women. Clearly the doctor knew all about it, had personal experience and presumably had said the same thing to many women. But I hadn't needed HRT up till then and I told him I wanted to keep going without it. Instead, I took up his suggestion of vaginal oestrogen pessaries, which I found easy to use, and sex became comfortable again.

Up till then, I hadn't thought about what life would be like during menopause. Neither my mother nor anyone else had talked about what happened after their last period. From what I had seen of Mum's experience and from gossip, I thought menopause involved only hot flushes, mood swings, and unreliable and possibly difficult periods followed by thinning bones. I had imagined that life would continue much as it had before but without the monthly rhythms and regular physical changes associated with periods. I didn't know that menopause was actually the time after my last period, when my ovaries stopped producing oestrogen and my body adjusted to hormonal changes. I was quite unprepared for what came next.

Over the months following my last period, there were a number of unwelcome signs as the effects of the change permeated my life in ways I had not envisaged. It affected my everyday capacity to function, my sex life and my appearance. It was the impact on my day-to-day ability to perform that was the most difficult to cope with. I often found it difficult to retain information. At the time I was attending evening lectures at university and I'd get halfway through writing down a sentence and find that I'd completely forgotten the second half.

I began to suffer from insomnia. I would lie in bed wide awake for hours, night after night. Some nights my legs would twitch uncontrollably. During the day at work, I felt light-headed and slightly nauseous, often talking in disjointed sentences and hoping nobody noticed. Eventually, I'd be so tired that I would crash and sleep through the night. But the pattern would soon start over.

As well as scratchy sex, my libido took a complete nosedive. That submerged giant, which is always with you, liable to rise up and overwhelm you at any time, had lain down and gone to sleep. It woke occasionally but not often. That sense of being possessed by a powerful force not just driving one's sex life but generating energy and a zest for tackling life had dissipated. Initially I felt its loss quite keenly, feeling that I had lost one part of my capacity to experience life intensely.

I understood osteoporosis and the effects of oestrogen loss on my bones, but I hadn't realised my hair and skin would also start to thin. My thick, full-bodied hair started to thin and look more like old lady's hair. My skin was losing its smooth suppleness. I was appalled to notice that my thighs were getting a lumpy, orange-peel look to them.

Martin said reassuringly that he couldn't see much change and they still looked pretty good to him. But I thought I was physically aging before my time. I was only forty-seven! I put on weight as my metabolism slowed down and I acquired a little pot of fat on my stomach.

My body thermostat didn't function properly either. I'd stopped having hot flushes but my body temperature seemed to bear no relation to the outside temperature. I often couldn't tell if the weather was warm or cold. But I did know when it was hot and developed intolerance to heat. I had noticed this coming on during my forties as my hormones started to wind down and it gradually got worse. This affected my bushwalking. Martin and I share a love for exploring and bushwalking, heading off on Sundays in the hills around our hometown of Melbourne and backpacking in Tasmania and parts of Australia's high country. The exercise and time spent in the bush created a feeling of physical and mental well-being that had given me a healthy perspective on the ups and downs of life. It kept me on an even keel – well, for most of the time. But I came to dread going walking when the temperature went over about twenty-seven degrees. I would quickly overheat, feel listless and very uncomfortable. Martin didn't understand this and thought I was making excuses to get out of a walk. 'Hot?' he'd say. 'It's not hot!' This was the only part of my menopause that caused marital friction. As soon as the temperature dropped, I was rearing to go. I often felt very lethargic doing things that I normally performed effort-lessly. I enjoy cycling and there is a short, easy hill near my home but instead of pedalling steadily, I sometimes had to get off and walk. Although I wasn't depressed in the clinical sense, I found depressing the thought that the rest of my life might continue like this. I felt that nature had chucked me on the scrapheap now that I'd lost my capacity to reproduce the species.

I didn't want to put up with feeling awful and decided to do something. I visited a women's health resource centre and borrowed a pile of books on menopause. There were books that advocated HRT as the only solution, others that stridently opposed it; advice on natural remedies for various symptoms; and discussions of the ostracism and taboos that surround women's bleeding. While the books were full of information, advice and opinions, I didn't find that they helped me to decide what I should do. There was no well-trodden path of women's wisdom to guide my way forward.

After about a year I decided to give HRT a go. Just as I didn't find all I wanted to know in the books I'd read, I also wasn't sure who to consult to canvas the full range of options. I had done enough reading to know that I wanted to use patches because the hormones bypass the digestive system and enter straight into the bloodstream. Unlike swallowing pills, this meant a lower dosage could be taken for the same effect. As an alternative to patches, I was prepared to discuss Livial, synthetic hormone pills, which a friend in England had been happily taking for a few years. However, in 1997 Livial was not available in Australia, nor were patches containing both oestrogen and progesterone. The GP who'd hinted at a great sex life on HRT had retired before I'd decided to give HRT a go. I had a high regard for the doctoring skills and empathy of the GP who'd replaced him. He prescribed an oestrogen patch which I changed twice a week, and daily progesterone tablets. I stopped using the vaginal oestrogen pessaries as they were not necessary when taking HRT.

The effect was almost immediate. I slept well, my little potbelly disappeared, my energy returned and I functioned like a normal member of the human race again. The only thing that didn't surge back was my libido. To get this back I would need to add testosterone to the cocktail. As our sex was still enjoyable and intercourse was no longer painful, I decided to do without this extra hormone.

I took HRT for five years and stopped in late 2002 when there was a lot of negative publicity in the media about the adverse effects of HRT. Over the previous two years the progesterone had been causing increasing tenderness in one of my breasts. I'd decreased my daily dose to taking it for two weeks out of every four, mimicking the menstrual cycle, which meant I started having monthly bleeds again. However, the breast tenderness continued and I was uneasy about taking something that gave me a constantly sore breast.

It was time to see if I could manage without it. I decided to give myself a break from HRT for three to four months and discussed this with my prescribing doctor. He supported my decision and told me to return if I had any problems. It was clear in my mind that if my symptoms returned and I could not manage I would go back onto some form of HRT.

It was not long before I was again spending long hours staring at a dark ceiling, well after the last trams for the night had ceased rumbling along the road. Within a fortnight I was feeling desperate again, eyes heavy, words trailing off halfway through sentences, forgetting what I was talking about.

I returned to my GP. He was always happy to talk about options for handling menopause and was open-minded on different treatments, pointing out that most of the treatments had been monitored for too short a period to know what really worked and what the long-term effects were likely to be. However, I felt that he treated menopause as just another medical problem. He didn't really understand the anxiety and uncertainty about the future that these physical and mental changes had created in me. Menopause is one of those things you have to experience first hand – or live with someone who is going through it – to really understand what it is like.

I felt trapped. Without HRT I was a mess, with HRT I had breast tenderness. The choices seemed bleak: feel awful or risk my health. I wanted to talk about what was happening to me and ask the advice of someone who knew what it was like. I decided to try the Women's Clinic at Melbourne's Royal Women's Hospital. To my horror I had to wait six weeks for an appointment. I could be insane by then! The delay turned out to be a blessing in disguise. By the time the date arrived I was sleeping better and none of my other symptoms had returned, though the little pudding basin of fat on my stomach was rebuilding itself.

At the hospital I had a long chat with a young woman doctor who told me rather depressingly that all my previous symptoms would return and that if I wasn't managing I should come back and see her to discuss what to do. Apart from telling me that I could have been taking a much lower dose of progesterone for the previous five years, she didn't give me any more comfort than my GP. It was clear that she was also not talking from experience and that she didn't really understand the dilemmas I was grappling with. Fortunately my previous symptoms didn't return. I think that during the five years of HRT my system must have settled down and adapted. In fact I felt pretty good. It is now four years later and I feel fit, healthy and full of energy.

I believe there were a number of things that helped me through menopause. Bushwalking and camping in remote places were physically invigorating and brought me peace of mind. Brisk walking and bike riding have been part of my life for years and I fit them in where I can as an alternative to driving. I kept these activities up even when I felt lacking in energy or overheated, I just popped a wet scarf around my neck to keep the heat down.

When insomnia started, I cut my caffeine intake to one luxurious coffee for breakfast and a couple of cups of tea during the day, none in the evening. I stretch and practise yoga, finding the exercises and relaxation routine effective for better sleep. The stretches also helped to stop my leg twitching. I still have occasional bouts of sleeplessness when nothing will work, but I know it will pass. I will always have to watch what I eat. No longer can I attack a large plate of food like a plague of locusts and I'm resigned to having a small potbelly. I read that abdomen fat is a source of oestrogen after menopause, so I think it is meant to be there.

The tenderness in my breast gradually disappeared after stopping HRT although I have had occasional soreness. It appears to be a bit of mastitis that I could have medicated if necessary. Mammograms and breast checks keep this monitored. My recent bone-density scan showed my bones are good, and the condition of my skin and hair are following normal patterns for my age. Intercourse didn't become painful again. My libido never returned but I have stopped missing it. The angst and intensity have been replaced by a serenity and a reflectiveness which yield a richness of feeling and experience that more than make up for what I lost when my libido vanished.

I have always been able to talk to my husband about what was happening to me and, apart from when he thought his beloved bushwalking was threatened, he has been very sympathetic to the tribulations of menopause. We both mourned the passing of my libido but our affection and physical intimacy has meant that our relationship has stayed rewarding, if lacking the heady passions of our youth.

I am enjoying my post-menopausal years. For me, life is very good.

Jenny retired from work at fifty-five. She enjoys writing, works in the community with refugees, spends more time with family and friends, and indulges her love of bushwalking and the outdoors.

Because Jenny's menopause started earlier than usual, her friends could not relate to her symptoms. She found it strange that women can talk to each other about periods but don't want to discuss menopause. Because of her experience, she listens, comforts and helps any woman who approaches her about menopause. Her wish is for menopause to become a publicly accepted rite of passage, like puberty.

LYNNE'S STORY (PART ONE)

I was overwhelmed and fascinated by Lynne's story. I didn't know how to make sense of it. As Lynne had written: 'How do you write about menopause? Is this where symptoms fit in? How do I tie it all together?' I put it down and picked it up again, drawn to her brilliant writing. I pulled her story apart and decided to make it two separate stories. I could relate to it all. And so will you.

I stand in the kitchen in stockinged feet and skirt and blouse
Hair washed, scraggy, still have to blow-dry.
Where's my watch? Fingers flicker through my bag
Wallet, glasses, driving glasses
Need the sheet about the dental health clinic, need to ring
    orthodontist.
Is the cat still inside, check heater is off, walk into bedroom
Thinking
Petrol, yes, okay, have to get the back tyres checked
Imagine having a flat in the middle of Belconnen Way at nine
    in the morning!
Visions of cars parked on the roadside, hazard lights flashing
Where is that on the car?
Will I take the blue shoes or wear the red?

Need to put my runners on for the walk from the car park
    to work.
Suck my stomach in and I haven't swum for two weeks
Standing in the bedroom
Thinking
Why am I here?
Fuck!
Turn around and walk back to kitchen
Pass Catherine's door, was she dressed warmly this morning?
Did the kids have their vitamins?
And dinner, what's in the fridge?
Take chicken out of freezer, leave on bench
Is it going to be okay all day out of the fridge, probably not.
Check milk, need bread
Did I turn the heater off?
Shit, it's five past and I've been late two days in a row.
Grab keys.
What did I forget?

Menopause does not necessarily mean memory loss, but
being a busy middle-aged woman and having obligations
does. And menopause goes with middle age. The whole
notion of moving from the kitchen to the bedroom and
sustaining the thought of why I was going there is no go.
But I have a theory. As we grow older there is so much
behind us, so much experience, so many facts stored away,
that the failure to recall some things is simply due to our
minds having to sift through so much more. So it takes
more time. I have no medical evidence to support my
theory, neither has it been rejected. This gets my theory to
first base and provides me with substantial relief.

I can still remember the day I first lost a word. It was 'match'. I could recall its size, colour, length, what it was made from, and could describe the little box it came in. But what was it called? When I finally asked someone, I then couldn't recall why I needed it. But as I said, my memory has a lot to sift through. And it was only a match.

I have been living alongside menopause for a number of years. Since my mid forties I started to see physical changes, felt emotional shifts, and I wondered, 'Is this a menopausal thing?' I sense things I cannot find words for. I don't know if that is part of menopause, or being middle-aged, or the complexity of this time in my life. Or perhaps it's woman-hood. I thought I could list my symptoms like going through adolescence, or pregnancy. I can't. There are so many layers to menopause. I can't just write about hot flushes or despair. I have to approach menopause as something organic, something that shifts and changes. Just as a growing body has to be considered alongside the psychological and emotional changes of adolescence, so menopause, too, needs to be handled while experiencing middle age with all its complications.

Strange moods. Different. I'm not sure if it is physiolog-ical or life accumulating, having more things to look back on, the result of fifty-two years of living. I have felt strange, bleak, dark and lonely, but also something else. I am aware of treading onto new ground, I see myself through others' eyes (my mother's eyes) and see disbelief. I feel shaky with this new awareness.

Menopause and growing into an older person intensi-fies my sense of who I am in terms of womanhood. In trying to understand the changes happening to me, I look at other women my age. I think back to when I was younger and how I perceived middle-aged women. When we are young we do not want to acknowledge that we, too, will grow old. I never really saw older women. I was patronising because they didn't have smooth skin and they had nothing to say I hadn't heard before. So where does all that put me now?

Menopausal changes and the realities of an aging body meant a gradual uncovering of my own preconceptions about the women I had grown up with, who'd preceded me, my own family and women at work or in the street. I learned that fixating on the changes is pointless. They will happen. I have accepted that part of the mid-life/ menopause journey is making the shift from a young woman getting older to an older woman in a different place.

On some level I find this journey, my physical changes, fascinating. Our faces and bodies are shaped by the lives, inner and outer, that we have so far lived. I find this an exciting thought, and a warning. I cannot hide behind my smooth skin and nice hair any more. Who I am is all out there. There is an exhausted frowning look my face settles into when I am deep in thought, and my face collapses into a wrinkled map of happiness when I see someone I love or reach for my children. I love old faces and admire graceful and serene older women – their beauty always speaks to me of something to be valued. In that way a sense of personal beauty has not disappeared from my life or the life of the beautiful women who are my friends and fellow travellers. I know that some people might think, 'Well, of course she would say that . . . poor thing.' I don't have the classic bone structure but I do have the laughter lines and the silver rivers in my hair.

I have developed the middle-aged woman walk. I know I have because I have noticed it in other women my age. It combines determined, energetic busyness with a sort of grounded weariness. There is bounce but nothing of the fluidity and slow, easy grace of young limbs. Is it a menopausal body reconfiguration? Or the fact that we are the maintenance people? We have to juggle many things at once and hence need to move fast. We feed people; we keep places safe and comfortable; we educate, pay, heal, protect, fix, clean, negotiate, replace, decide, transport, deliver, and we do it on several different fronts day after day. So we walk fast.

At the same time as I was going through all the changes associated with menopause, I noticed that I was becoming increasingly invisible to men. It was a relief. Unwanted attention from men is not pleasant, talking to a man and seeing that sudden shift in his eyes which means he is looking at me as a woman and not a work colleague or someone to chat to on the bus. Not all women feel as I do on this. I like men and the different view they have on things, but attraction needs to be mutual.

Not only am I not noticed much these days by men, women, children, teachers and shop staff, I am not taken seriously. Perhaps this is not a new problem for me because I have always had to make an effort to be seen and heard. I think it's because I am short and do not have a strong physical presence. I have a decreased ability to endure fools. I get more annoyed than I used to. I don't put up with as much shit. I don't know if this is menopausal moodiness or finally coming to my senses. I am impatient with dishonesty, slowness that is not justified, people who try to distract me from my path, children who will not do as they are asked, adults who don't deliver when they say they will. I used to make excuses for people. Not any more.

I noticed this shift, for the first time, when I had to speak to my son's teacher about him being put into a class for slow readers. In a patient, long-suffering voice the teacher told me that in his opinion my son was barely literate and that it was not unusual for parents to be surprised, and so on. For years this behaviour reduced me to a cringing, apologetic I know you're a busy, professional, can't-go-wrong, caring person, and I am just another silly, time-wasting, annoying parent who knows nothing. Not any more. I sat facing the teacher and felt a twinge of anticipation for confrontation that was new and quite pleasing. In my new middle-aged self-awareness, I have developed two approaches. Both are motherly. There is the sudden, sharp outrage followed by something positive, like a verbal pat on the head for being a good teacher; and there is the smiling, motherly, bloody-minded persistence. On that occasion I felt calm when asking, how could a boy who has completed reading *Lord of the Rings* be backward in reading?

Menopause is more than physical and emotional changes. It's part of a continuum. I look not only toward where I am going but also from where I have come. The future is different, it's full of older people when it used to be filled with young and old, the past is richer, there is more there, and I am in all of it. Yet I still hold the newness of those things.

Experiences the young are just going through I remember experiencing, over and over, as a child, a teenager, young woman, new mother, as a worker. I look at older women and wonder about them. They are unknown territory. If I have had to make major internal readjustments with the unfolding reality of middle-age, then I also have to face my preconceptions about being sixty, seventy, eighty. I have become aware of my own greater inner complexity, encompassing a range of acquired skills and knowledge and experience so vast that I no longer have easy access to all that I know. There are levels of intuitive and emotional knowledge that I don't quite understand but know it is best not to ignore. So what of those who are ahead of me, where must they be behind those eyes?

Just as I feel a special responsibility for young women so I look to older women and know they know things I have yet to discover. I look at the faces of women in their sixties and realise there's more to come. It's not finished yet!

LYNNE'S STORY (PART TWO)

There is something about menopause and female friends. Is this a menopausal thing or a woman thing? There is a necessity for the company of women. We share exhaustion, sleepless nights, damp clothes, anxiety and confusion. We talk about hairy chins, daughters and sons, discontent, diets, wrinkles, and other women. The conversation stops when a man enters the room. We don't miss a beat when a daughter enters. Our daughters stand back with silent, piercing eyes or drape themselves over us and look and sometimes listen and always learn. We laugh at them without saying why. We snap and poke them with our fingers, daring the ones who will follow us. Our eyes meet and when they do it's all open. The experiences we share are on emotional and physical levels; things we are going through now, and things we remember from our youth that our daughters are going through.

My daughter is on a mattress on the floor drawing, and watching Dr Who. *Her friend sits behind her on the couch. I have asked my girl to talk to her friend, who could be bored. They both object but her friend's face is looking at neither my daughter nor the TV show. I am aware that sometimes things must be left to unfold as they will.*

Her mother arrives and I offer her coffee, but she can't stay. Her son is waiting in the car, waiting for his mother to take him to soccer. Her daughter reluctantly gathers up her things. We talk quickly, catching up on each other's news. When she leaves, we say we must try to find time for lunch but we know lunch will constantly fall over in the face of cooking, housework, children, appointments, unexpected happenings. The phone rings, something boils over on the stove, and my daughter rushes to the bathroom. I know why. It's that time of the month.

When my periods became sporadic I went to see a doctor who suggested hormone treatment. Along with the prescription, she gave me a list of the possible side effects. I read through them and decided they were worse than what I was going through at the time so decided to treat HRT as a backstop. Much later, when my last period lasted for thirty days, I went to another doctor, weak, desperate and scared. He prescribed the pill, ignoring my fears even though I was visibly pale and shaky from loss of blood. My period stopped two weeks later and never returned. I didn't feel any loss of womanhood; I have three children and my periods gave me hell every month for thirty-five years. I hated them from the start.

I have always looked at health holistically for myself and my children, using traditional medicine only when all else failed or the ailment involved antibiotics or stitches. So far, and it's been about seven years, I have been able to manage my menopause using vitamin and herbal supplements, exercise, diet, and stress-relief techniques. I read self-help books and anything I can find on menopause. I've tried different things. I stop when I feel they no longer work. I tried soy milk but it gave me stomach pains. I bought some tofu but the kids refused to touch it. Currently, I'm using a lovely cream with wild yam, geranium, sage oil and linseed. It's a pleasure just to read the ingredients. Now and then I take evening primrose because it has a small effect on my mood and I love the name.

My teenage son is still in his pyjamas though it is gone lunchtime. He worries me, his lack of exercise, his laziness. I am sick of yelling at him and he fights back better. Or as a male? I am aware of the importance of space and of my difficulty in letting go. Of my fear for his happiness. Of his future that I can't clearly see. It is the same with my daughter. Sometimes all I can do is keep them fed and warm. I know that no matter what I do they are going to feel pain and loss, and no matter what I think I am always going to feel I could have done better.

The fact that menopause and middle age happen side by side is relevant. Because all of my body is aging, diet and exercise are very important. They affect my energy levels, strength and flexibility, my immunity to illness, and they also have an effect on my moods, both immediately and days later. I don't eat as well as I should but this is a deliberate decision. When I see the misery and hunger there is in the world, I can't see the point of not celebrating the riches I was blessed with living in Australia. I try to eat what I should as well as what I want rather than cut back on the things I like. If I get a bit heavy, I increase the healthy food as this fills me up so there is little room for the not so healthy stuff. I avoid all processed food for my family and me. Except Cherry Ripes and Drumsticks!

I make my son have a shower, do a job for me and have a bit of exercise before going on the computer. He whines. He doesn't want to ride his bike and says he will go for a walk. Exercise when you can, menopausal thing; mother/son thing, find things to do together you both like. I ask if I can walk with him knowing he will grumble, but he says yeah. He criticises me all the way because

I walk more than a block and he has his slippers on. We talk of other things and he says, yeah, right. I try to explain something and he says, yeah, whatever Mum. I ask him to pick me a branch of flowing gold and orange autumn leaves and he says he hates orange and am I going to do this all the way. Then he jumps up and pulls off a neon-lit branch. I say I knew he was good for something. There is a lengthy, worrying silence. I didn't mean that I add and he groans, yeah I know. Then there is sweetness in the silence.

I swim and walk whenever I can. I don't actually swim, I dog paddle, breaststroke or lie on my back and kick my legs, anything that will keep me moving forward. I do yoga at home when I feel stiff, especially around my back and legs. I do these things at my own pace. I am not precious or self-judging about my exercise. I'm not athletic enough and it might stop me from doing it.

While I am walking with my son I become aware of the power of pausing, waiting, listening, sharing. I am tempted to call it menopause because 'pause' is something that is part of it. I look up to my seventeen-year-old son, full of adolescence. I am his fifty-two-year-old menopausal mum. There is a parallel between adolescent angst and menopausal madness. In my deepest heart I feel wilder and less respecting of the tidy world I inhabit and maintain, and inflict on him. We share this feeling and we both have a sense of humour that is warm and silly.

Migraines are part of my menopause. My migraines started before I knew what they were and before I was aware of my own menopause. Because of my weak eyes, headaches have always been a part of my life. In my mid forties, however, I had a headache that reduced my life to a small, hot, screaming place which needed a house call from a doctor and an injection that knocked me out. I had another migraine, and another. I was all pain. I couldn't think or talk or act. I curled up on the floor, behind closed curtains, a blanket covering me, veering away from sunlight, sharp-edged, razor-fingered. After the third migraine I realised this was a problem that might not go away. I visited the doctor and received a prescription for a pill to be taken half-hourly. When I started this treatment, the effect didn't kick in until the third pill, by which time I'd reached a screaming crescendo of pain.

I don't understand migraines. I have talked to other women and have learnt that for each the migraine is different. Remedies and management, too, are different. After two years of trial and error and much pain I found that lavender oil dabbed around my temples combined with taking Panadol works. I do not go anywhere without these. For others, it doesn't work. And for all migraine sufferers, keeping out of the light and staying still are essential, until a bearable level is reached.

I am in the kitchen washing the dishes. My son walks in to tell me there is something on the radio about migraines. We misunderstand each other, as usual, and I ask what did it say? and he says it's just a short thing, a few minutes and I ask again, but what did it say? He says turn the radio on and walks out. I turn on the radio in the kitchen and realise that it is a program in progress, not something he heard. A woman from Kenya speaks of her migraines. A woman doctor cites links between oestrogen levels and migraine, exercise and migraine; how it's different for everyone; how ordinary painkillers can work if the timing is right, but not for everyone; about the inability to work and stopping to throw up on the side of the road (yes!). I know these things but I'm amazed at the coincidence. I am amazed that my son came in to tell me about it. I feel a deep sense of accomplishment as a mother and a sweetness of pleasure at how nice a boy he is.

During my menopause my body shape and texture were changing in ways I knew were irreversible, some things unexpected. Initially I felt sad at the loss of my golden smooth thighs, calm unlined face, thick hair with its rainbow highlights, and platform stomach. There is a sponge where my middle used to be and I have folds of loose skin on my back. An S-bend wraps around my stomach, thighs, hips and bum that arrived one morning and has never gone away.

I love my hands. They are bony and the veins are large and blue. The skin is fine and finely lined. Like crepe, papery thin. In my menopausal years they are the part of my body I value most. They can do so much. They are skilled, delicate, strong. I can heal with a touch, avert disaster, console and create. There is a history of learning and accomplishment from many failures overcome. They have a practical grace, sliding through air like silk, every moment a caress.

My hands are picking up litter at the front of our house and I wish the kids would help me. But I don't ask because I can't be bothered with the hassle. I walk into the kitchen, my hands holding bits of paper and plastic, a crushed Coke tin and a cigarette packet. You haven't started smoking again, my son gives me an accusing look. No, I say, annoyed he has jumped on me. I dump the rubbish into the bin and wash my hands under running warm water with ti-tree-oil soap. I dry them, noticing that my knuckles are red and slightly enlarged. I stroke the pale brown splotches that cover my hands and set them to work peeling potatoes.

Hair grew in new places and disappeared from others. I was surprised by hairs on my chin, strong and wiry and dark, and totally unprepared for them appearing on my neck. In retrospect I realise there have always been hairy middle-aged women around me but I believed it was because they were naturally like that. Hair on my head is thinning. Every morning I have to deal with a comb full of lost hair, it is now only about a third of what it used to be. This is a mixed blessing. My hair was extremely thick, fine and straight and prone to doing its own thing, so having less is easier to manage. But it feels strange and, though I like my patchwork of silver and brown streaks, I miss the sense of luxury and the soft richness.

Hot flushes are definitely part of my menopause. I have had fevers before but hot flushes are not like that. I am suddenly overcome with a heat and there is a strong sense of disorientation. It is particularly disconcerting if I am talking to someone at the time and suddenly I am burning and nothing around me has changed. When the waves recede, and I am back to where I was before the heat, some time has passed and the world has moved on, without me. This is also disconcerting. That abrupt withdrawal is more disturbing for me than the hot flush.

But more distressing than hot flushes, is this undercurrent of despair I seem to live with and which is part of these years. It's not madness I feel. I feel lost. I have done a lot of the things I set out to do, failed and succeeded; and seen unexpected consequences. But what now? I can't go back to where I was before and I don't want to. While I am still learning, experiencing and growing, a fundamental change is happening in my body, mind and soul. It's still me, but I am living in a body that is aging and demanding more attention from me. It's like I am in mid flight and need to change direction. But to where? What do I want? The obvious things, yes, like financial security, healthy kids, happiness and space to write. Every so often I sense a clear, peaceful certainty and then I start to panic again until I am hauled out by another part of me which stands, arms folded, and says, 'Just get on with it, will you!' I look back now and see how huge the journey has been, how far-reaching and intricate. Like an old piece of lace I feel delicate, parts finely wrought and marvellously imaginative, parts frayed at the edges and thin with wear. I am growing in a different way, weighed and shaped by the past and I have an urgent new strength and energy, a vision and insight emerging amidst new aches and sadnesses and sudden, strange despairs.

I am in the kitchen and my hands are pulling together the pieces for dinner. I can do that, pull the pieces together instead of painstakingly following a recipe. It's the result of years spent in the kitchen, years of handling food, feeding people. The kitchen resonates through my years, a place of anxiety and stress, exhaustion, tedium, comfort, skill, achievement, pleasure. Love. It's women's equivalent of the shed. My son wanders in and picks at the ingredients. I say, stop it. But he grins and shoves chunks of cheese into his mouth. I snap, there'll be none left. He laughs and pats me clumsily, towering over me as if I am a small furry animal. I am immensely happy.

Lynne is a librarian and works at the University of Canberra. She is completing a postgraduate diploma in Professional Writing and is a single mother of three children, with two still at home. Her priorities are her children, her writing and her job – in that order.

ON BEING INVISIBLE

Canberra Uni is full of short, round middle-aged women
    like me
Standing with our coffee, books, bag and key
Balanced on a wall with our tidy lips, tidy hands, eyes that see
    everything
Or walking through car-park rain
Complacent, compact, complete
The only one with an umbrella
And in our cars Band-Aids, disprin, a torch with batteries
    and working
Matches, a full first-aid set in the glove compartment.
Middle-aged women have low, slow voices,
Our words spread to each corner, I have seen you look, check,
    move on.
We have taught you politeness and attention,
Around us it occurs to you to do right,
Universal mothers, grandmothers, aunts, big sisters
Behave, get it right, we insist in our tidy tidy places.
But deep down flickering, errant, a secret hunger darts.
I want to swear (without apology)
I hate these ugly clothes that bind and contain and fade
I want to wear peacock blue and feathers
And a cat at my feet and butterflies around my head

And rivers of pearls from my earlobes
Be real and filled with my years
Intensely me, rooted to the earth
Head embracing the stars, sun dissolving in my blood.
But perhaps not, and I flow, ebb, recede again
With lowered head I move on.
To do more would upset the children.
Annoy the men. And we really don't want that.

Rhonda Cotsell

DIERDRE'S STORY

Dierdre and her husband have been married for thirty years and have worked together in their own business for most of their marriage. They have two daughters who have recently completed their education away from home at Monash University in Victoria. Dierdre admits that she and her husband found the departure of their daughters very difficult to handle. They felt lost and threw themselves into their work to fill in the empty space that was now in their lives. It was towards the end of their daughters' first year of university that Dierdre's menopause started.

My menopause arrived unexpectedly when I was forty-seven. The symptons could not have arrived at a more inopportune time. I had been married for twenty-five years and our relationship was going through that taking-each-other-for-granted stage. We were both experiencing the 'empty nest' syndrome and in an odd way we felt like two strangers without our children around us any longer. Because we worked together our conversation was always about business and we were out of touch with talking about personal issues, particularly emotions. We both needed support but had lost the knack and we just let things drift.

Our two daughters were both away from home undertaking degrees at Monash University and their departure changed the dynamics of our lives. Of course we were proud of their successes and thrilled to see them venturing down their own paths. They started uni at the same time so we didn't lose one daughter and then the other later, which may have better prepared us for our new 'childless' marriage. Our eldest daughter worked for nearly two years after high school before starting her degree, but our youngest didn't want a break between school and uni and they were both keen to leave together, supporting each other.

We had had twenty-one years of ballet, netball, tennis and a short-term infatuation with horse riding; school committees, fundraising for everything from balls to halls; worry over chicken pox, a broken arm, tantrums, failed driving test, four pets including a dog that killed the lizard; and so forth. Our lives revolved around our girls – their happiness, their education and development. It's not unusual. And it was wonderful, neither of us would have had it any other way. But now they were gone.

Al and I are both architects and we have had our own small business for over fifteen years. We design home additions, carports, pergolas and manage the construction of our work. For the first few years we operated from home which was fantastic for us and the girls. Then, for professional reasons, we leased an office and we continue to run the business from there.

So, at forty-seven, my girls left and started university interstate. As well as struggling with this I started a new phase in my life – menopause. My periods had never been regular and when three months passed with no sign of them I didn't take much notice. Frankly, I was glad when they didn't appear. I was always reduced to curling up into a foetal position clutching a hot-water bottle for the first couple of hours. Pain would gnaw my back, hips, stomach and thighs. Panadol was my only friend. In that first year of my menopause I sometimes skipped a month, some months it was a normal cycle and other times I just had a bit of spotting.

I knew I was menopausal when the hot flushes started. They were fierce and fiery. I'd burn up to the point where I felt I was going to ignite and then, just as suddenly, I'd cool down and freeze. There was no way I could hide them or fob them off as feeling a bit hot because I would be drenched, with wet hair sticking to my scalp, wet clothes clinging to my breasts and, if a skirt, stuck around my bum and legs. Winter or summer, it made no difference and when I went to bed I had a fan whirling all night. There had been some very embarrassing times at work so I started to take a change of clothes with me and I even had my hair cut short so I didn't have limp strands falling around my face.

Al knew I was menopausal but neither of us knew for how long these flushes would continue. There were times when I was having them every half an hour. I decided to see a doctor and our very large medical centre had about twenty doctors. Although my regular doctor was a male I thought a female doctor might be better. I telephoned the centre. 'Could you please tell me who are your female doctors and how old they are?' I asked.

'I beg your pardon?' the receptionist said and I asked again their ages. She said she wasn't sure but thought Dr A was about thirtyish, Dr B mid forties, and Dr C sixty.

'I'll take the sixty-year old,' I said, and explained that I was menopausal and wanted to talk to a woman who had been through it.

When I arrived for my appointment I told the doctor of my severe hot flushes and I asked her in what other ways menopause might affect me. To my surprise, rather than discuss this, she typed in 'menopause' on her computer and, after some time finding the right site, read out a list of symptoms. I said that I had already searched the internet and had the list of symptoms but could she enlighten me with more information. She asked me if I wanted to go onto HRT. I said, 'No, I do not want to go onto HRT,' more out of annoyance than from an informed decision. I was disappointed that she gave no indication of personal understanding and, whether it was my imagination or not, I thought she seemed slightly embarrassed. I had also wanted to discuss with her (the whole reason for seeing a female) my complete disinterest in sex these days. I thought it might be something to do with the flushes as I couldn't bear to be close to my husband and I was making excuses to avoid any physical contact with him. I got no further than saying that I wanted to talk about another matter when she said that my time had run out and that I should make another appointment. I was flabbergasted.

I drove home quite distressed. It wasn't until the following morning that Al remembered to ask how I went at the doctor's but I just brushed passed him with a pile of files under my arm and shouted that I had to go on HRT. We had been trying hard to adjust to our new situation without the girls and I soon realised that our conversations were about two things: the girls and work. We had talked about little else for years. Al was a bit reserved when it came to talking about personal things, particularly on an emotional front. He could talk about business and discuss designs with clients and builders until the cows came home. He was very work focused and could be intolerant when dealing with people issues.

The week following my visit to the doctor was very tense between us. Al ignored me and expected me to sort myself out. Although I knew this was only his way, I felt frustrated and angry that he was not taking an interest in my predicament. We had been good partners in work and as parents, but when it came to personal things, I knew I couldn't rely on Al for comforting words and tender support. I had known this since I met Al, and it had never bothered me. But now I felt vulnerable and in need of loving care. Al didn't know how to respond to my needs and I didn't know how to ask. When my daughters had been at home I would flop onto their bed and listen to their troubles with boys or their concern with skin blemishes. We would laugh together over a hair colour gone wrong and cry together over the break-up with a boyfriend. But I didn't have them around me now and text messages are just not the same. In their place I had menopause.

In addition to the profuse sweating, I started to experience nausea. At first I thought it was food poisoning, but then a friend said she had the same thing and that nausea often accompanied hot flushes. I felt quite desperate. I had picked up several brochures on menopause and ticked off only three on the long list of symptoms: severe hot flushes, nausea and loss of libido. However, only having three didn't make me feel any better. I decided to make an appointment with a naturopath because I had to do something to control my flushes. I tried progesterone cream but it made little difference. I took a course of black cohosh, dong quai and wild yam plus vitamins C and E, but again the relief was not sufficient.

The night sweats and loss of libido really affected us. Any closeness with Al made me feel hot and claustrophobic. My vagina was dry and intercourse painful, so I gave no encouragement to have sex. For the first time in my life I was experiencing cystitis after intercourse. Burning pain and rushing to the toilet every ten minutes to urinate would go on for days. I felt abused and in my head blamed my discomfort on Al.

However, my pain was not as bad as Al's. I had no idea at the time, but he suspected me of having an affair. Considering my avoidance of anything intimate and our lack of personal communication and understanding of menopause, it was a reasonable conclusion. We were so wrapped up in our own turmoil, both hurting, yet we avoided giving each other comfort. We drifted further apart.

I made an appointment with my usual (male) doctor, ready to try anything. I poured my heart out to him and he quietly nodded and murmured and waited for me to finish. He suggested patches of HRT and I willingly agreed. I tried the patches for two months but got little relief. I was very disappointed and thought I was doomed indefinitely. When I returned to the doctor he said that he could increase the dosage of the patches or prescribe HRT pills. I opted for the pills. The effect was almost immediate. My flushes ceased, the nausea stopped, and my periods returned – which I wasn't too pleased about. My body was working again. After about a fortnight I realised that the

flushes and nausea had also made me exhausted, something I had attributed to work and worry. I slept like a
sixteen-year-old, some nights ten hours straight. I ran
around like a young girl during the day and one Saturday
morning I went shopping and bought new clothes. It was
as if I couldn't bear to wear my 'hot flush' clothes any
longer. I phoned some girlfriends to arrange lunch, leaving
our office for a couple of hours—something I rarely did.
I was feeling wonderful. But all was not well with Al. He
was cold. I wanted him to feel happy with me and couldn't
understand why he was driving me away. I tried to talk to
him but he was awkward and I never liked to push him
when he was like that.

Unfortunately, HRT did not return my libido and
although my vagina seemed to be slightly better lubricated
it was still too dry for comfortable sex. I spoke to my
doctor who again listened attentively and nodded with
understanding. I was expecting him to prescribe some
magic potion and although he recommended any of the
personal gels or lubricating creams that you can buy from
the chemist, he suggested I talk to Al. My face must have
dropped because he asked how Al was coping with my
changes. I felt like screaming, 'Who the hell cares about Al's
feelings? I'm the one going through these changes.' But it
was only a fleeting thought because I really did care. My
doctor continued in his careful, quiet way and talked about
other ways to be intimate—oral sex and sexual aids, massage
and cuddles. There was a part of me that felt acutely embarrassed but my doctor was genuine and professional and I listened. Then he said that if I thought counselling might
help, he could recommend a doctor for Al and me to see. I
thought, you must be kidding—get Al to see a counsellor!

During the next semester break our daughters came home. It coincided with my fiftieth birthday. They had spoken to Al and wanted to prepare a surprise party for me. Poor Al had to go along with it. He didn't feel in a party mood. He had a happier wife on HRT but with no interest in sex (with him, he thought). I was told that we were going to dinner and to the Australian Ballet. We arrived at the Hyatt for dinner and I walked into a private room to be greeted by all my family and friends. I was thrilled to have my girls with me and to see friends I hadn't seen for years. Al put on a brave face but I felt his misery.

When we got home we couldn't talk because we had the girls with us. Ten days went by before the girls returned to uni and, oddly enough, I could hardly wait to get them out the door. The strain between Al and me was unbearable. I wanted to shake him, even scream at him. For the first time in our marriage, a marriage I had seen lasting forever, I panicked at the thought of it breaking up. But I didn't plunge into an hysterical outburst. I let a day pass and tried to think sensibly. In the end, Al and I were thinking as one. Just as I was going to broach the subject he, uncharacteristically, started first by asking me point blank if I was having an affair. I was gobsmacked! My hesitation only confirmed in his mind that I was. I could see him slipping out of my life and blurted out that it was ridiculous, that I had never even thought of having an affair, let alone wanted one. I was so emphatic and in his eyes I saw relief. Slowly he explained what he had believed. I sat on the lounge chair and listened to his anguish and realised, for the first time, that menopause had affected us both. We talked for a long time, talked about my visits to the doctor and his suggestions. Al listened calmly, said he didn't think we needed counselling but agreed with me that we needed to be a lot more open with our feelings.

It's hard to break a lifetime of habits and we easily fell into our old routine of just talking about work and what the girls were up to. Initially it was up to me to start the conversation on personal things that I thought were bothering us. Gradually Al grew less self-conscious but sometimes he would not respond and once again start to walk away. But I wouldn't let it drop.

We have been quite successful in our business, but the industry is very tough and our margins get less each year. I would like us to get out of the business or go smaller to reduce the long hours and stress. I know that I cannot handle the pressure any longer and I can see that Al is struggling with it too, although he would never admit it. I am sure that men, too, go through a 'change' in their middle years. There is less fun in Al these days and it takes a bit of effort to get him out of the office to do some 'living'. Over the past few years he has put on too much weight and is finding it difficult to change his diet and cut down on the beer. But he's aware of the health issues attached to his weight. It's something we talk about quite easily now, without him feeling embarrassed or me feeling like I am picking on him. He knows I genuinely care.

We are learning the importance of listening and talking, caring about and supporting each other's personal issues. It's new ground for us. I now realise Al is the most important person in my life. I am still on HRT and menopause is still part of my life. It's all part and parcel of aging issues. I know that I will come off HRT soon; I've been on it for three years and would like to be free of it. It's the little niggles in the back of my mind about the side effects, the unknown, and the stigma of HRT. When I told a thought-less friend I was on HRT, she responded, 'Oh, weren't you coping? Or is it vanity?'

She was one of the lucky women who hardly noticed menopause.

Dierdre and Al recently returned from a cruise in Scandinavia. It was the first holiday they have had in their marriage without their daughters.

With their degrees finished, their daughters are planning to live and work in Melbourne. Although Dierdre and Al were initially disappointed they accepted their daughters' decision better than they thought they would. The empty space left by the girls has now been filled by a concerted and willing effort on Dierdre's and Al's part to make their marriage happy.

When she weans herself off HRT Dierdre knows that some of her old menopause symptoms may return. 'If I do go through a rough patch, I know Al will give me support, and that is just as important as any drug – medical or natural,' she said.

BRONWYN'S STORY

Bronwyn has been a fitness instructor nearly all her adult life. Her classes include aerobics, yoga and special exercises for the elderly. She has worked all over Australia in gyms, schools, community centres and church halls, and now lives in the Northern Territory. Bronwyn's menopause started just before her fiftieth birthday and her main concerns have been the affect on her muscles and joints.

'Morning everyone, how are you all today?' I say to my class and walk over to turn the fans on. 'What a stinker of a weekend! Didn't quite reach forty degrees but it's going to today. We'll take it a bit easier this morning,' and I make the heat my excuse, but I'm thinking of the muscle pain in the lumbar region of my back and in my hips. I switch the fans on low. 'Is that okay or do you want more blast?' The class elects for a higher speed; they are already wilting. I select a CD of music that encourages a slower pace for the warm-up.

I am a fitness instructor. I've been teaching for the past thirty years and I love my job. I do all sorts of classes and there are some fancy names for them. There is Balance, Core, Tone, Sculpt, Cardio Blast, Fat Burner and Lite and Low. In the seventies we had Aerobics for Beginners, Intermediate and Advanced. Nothing elaborate about those names. But the leotards back then! They were amazing. Brilliant colours and designs, all with matching tights and leg warmers. As I look around my class this morning, the attire is cotton tees and loose-fitting shorts.

It wasn't until the mid 1980s that one had to be accredited to be a fitness leader. I was very supportive of this move. Before accreditation anyone could take an aerobics class, as long as they looked good and were fit. A lot of injuries were sustained in those days. I was one of the first to be professionally qualified.

I strap my microphone around me and walk to the front. 'Okay, let's do it! Warming up through the legs. Forward, three, two, one; and back. Again.' We move our limbs to the music and repeat several movements to warm up our muscles. I look at my class, checking that each person is moving properly. A small class today, all regulars and all women, except for Mario. He's solid and stocky and can usually be found in the gym lifting weights, but because his flexibility is almost zero he comes to my classes and he tries hard to loosen his knotted hamstrings and calves. 'Rolling the shoulders back, nice and slowly. And roll forward.' We prepare the body for a workout by increasing muscle temperature in each muscle group. 'Two steps to the side and back. Repeat to the left. Keep your breathing deep and even. Now grapevine to the right.' Ouch! My right hip muscle is as tight as a rock this morning. The pain kept me awake for hours last night. At least the left hip isn't quite as bad as it was last week. 'And grapevine to the left.'

The way aerobics is taught these days is vastly different to all those years ago when I started. Thank God! If we still did star jumps, high kicks and all that high-impact stuff that we did back then, I don't think I'd still be teaching. It's nothing to do with me not being fit enough. But it is to do with menopause.

I started getting muscle pain in my back and hips when I started menopause. I had my last period when I was around fifty years old. I'd always had regular periods and they'd never been a problem, except for the monthly pain which was like a hot football turning around and around in my stomach. It was when my periods stopped that I experienced severe muscle pain along with moderate pain in my joints. My hot flushes occurred mainly at night but they were not really bothersome. Accompanying the flushes were sleepless nights with unusual tiredness.

I sometimes wonder if getting these symptoms related to the end of my relationship with Tom. We'd been together for many years but agreed to separate. We are still friends and I have much admiration and respect for him. It does seem a coincidence that when we settled everything I started menopause. I didn't think I was under any undue stress, but perhaps it was there and my ovaries decided to retire. Guess they had to some time!

'Right leg forward, flex the foot back and slowly stretch.' I can hardly bend from the waist this morning, and all the muscles in my lower back hurt and are unyielding. I glance up from my bent position and catch Janet's face. 'And a little lower, if you can.'

I've never smoked and I think I'm healthier and fitter than the average person for my age. Well, let's be honest, I should be! When my menopause started to affect me I initially tried to find a solution with naturopathy. I wasn't keen to go on HRT, not without trying alternatives first. I was given progesterone cream for the muscle pain. I'd rub the cream on one part of my body, either my chest, behind my knees, triceps, stomach or inner thighs, changing to a different area each night. I persevered for about a year, the dose being changed a couple of times to give me better results. It helped a little and may be quite effective for some women with perhaps less muscle pain, but I really needed something else.

'Okay guys, get a drink while I change the tape,' I say to the class, rubbing my hip. I walk over to Janet and say, 'Hi Janet. Are you alright? You look really hot, before we've even got started.' Janet is fifty-nine and still has hot flushes. She gives me that anxious look—you know the one that says, 'How long is this going to go on for?' She says she is flushing every ten minutes lately and I advise her to keep her water bottle close by and sip regularly.

The pain I experienced in my muscles was very intense. It wasn't an ache and it wasn't a burning or shooting pain. It was a tight, hard pain. And it limited my mobility. I had never experienced anything like it before menopause. The constant pain kept me awake at nights and the lack of sleep was causing mild headaches, confusion and forgetfulness during the day. I started to take Valerian, a natural aid to help sleep, which I'd bought from the health food store. I also tried a cream that claims to be a herbal harmonising cream. Unfortunately neither helped me.

The music is more upbeat and I demonstrate the first move-ment. I make sure that all exercises are kind on the joints with flowing movements. And it's not just a physical workout but a mental one too! 'That's great guys, you're moving well.' The muscles and joints around my knees are also sore. I breathe deeply and move through the pain. No one would notice the agony I am in.

I never let on that I am in pain; I just work through it. When I am taking a class my whole focus is on the people in front of me: keeping the class engaged, at the appropriate level of difficulty, watching and observing each person to ensure that exercises are done correctly. And I love what I do. I shut out the pain and make my classes as enjoyable as possible for everyone. I talk all the way through.

Twenty-five years ago I would enthuse about the latest band on the scene or hot fashions, like platform shoes and flares. My classes seem to have grown older with me, and now we talk about aches and stiffness, fat bits here and flabby bits there.

My muscle and joint pain is not arthritis. When I turned fifty and menopause kicked in I went along to have a bone-density scan, thinking mine should be brilliant. But it showed 'average'. They tested the hip and lumbar. I immediately started on calcium supplements with added magnesium and various other minerals and trace elements. I took this for a year and went back for another bone-density scan. My hip density had increased by over one per cent and my lumbar density increased by five per cent, a significant improvement.

'Make sure your knees are aligning over your toes, Mario.' He checks himself and gives me a nod. 'That's better.' I give Janet a quick understanding smile. She appears to be having another hot flush; she's drenched, poor thing.

I have had the same masseuse for the past fourteen years. She knows my body very well – the pre-menopause body and the menopause body. It was Leah, my masseuse, who eventually convinced me that I should try HRT. The pain in the muscles and joints of my hips, lumbar and knees had reached the severe stage. She said that in her professional experience, HRT would make my muscles softer, less prone to injury and it would promote healing. Since being menopausal I have had two major muscle injuries: a hamstring tear (from yoga of all things) which took at least eight months to heal; and a shoulder injury (from playing golf) which took ten months to heal. Other symptoms I was experiencing were the crawling feelings under my skin around my knees and calves, flushes, confusion and forgetfulness. I was worried how these symptoms of menopause might affect my life and work and for how long. Sometimes, when I reflected on what was happening to my body I felt a wave of sadness wash over me and would be quite melancholy. I still feel this way.

I gave a lot of thought to Leah's recommendation of HRT and, with some trepidation, I chose quality of life over health issues.

I notice that half the class is struggling and the other half is rearing to go. This happens when I work in small communities; I get all sorts of fitness levels and I can change direction as quickly as a Darwin cyclone. 'For those who want to push harder, watch me now,' and I demonstrate a more challenging version. 'For the rest, follow me,' and I elect to do the easier steps to save my knees. 'Just work at your own pace.'

The first course of HRT I took was known as the 'discontinuous' HRT, which meant that I would still have periods. The GP I saw said that some women really like a bleed. I thought what a weird thing to say but when my periods finally stopped, I did feel that I had lost something. Quite recently, a very close aunt and my dog, Alf, had passed away and I thought, now another stage of my life has gone. I felt a bit unwomanly without a period – but I certainly didn't miss having a good bleed!

I took this HRT in tablet form for about four months but it was not satisfactory for me. From the onset I was having periods every nine days and with the regular loss of blood I was feeling light-headed and dizzy. The doctor changed the prescription to 'continuous' HRT and the periods stopped and never returned.

Leah was right. She noticed an improvement in my muscles within a week. I started to feel relief after five weeks. The pain in my muscles was gone, they were softer. It was bliss. However, as the months passed, I experienced little nagging doubts about the effects of HRT. After a little less than a year I decided to see if I could live without HRT. All the muscle pain returned as well as insomnia. I was in agony with my back and hips and returned to HRT and I have not dared to go off it since.

The whole class is working hard and I walk around encouraging individuals and correcting where necessary. The piece of music ends and I return to the front to change the CD for sit-ups and stretches. 'Fantastic, guys. Well done,' I say and give them a clap. 'Go and get a drink and bring back a mat for some floor work.' The class wanders off, grabbing water bottles, towels and mats. We stand for a few more minutes, cooling down, stretching calf muscles, hips, back and arms. 'Everyone okay?' and they respond with nods. 'Lying down, knees bent, feet hip width apart. You can put your arms across your chest or here or here,' I demonstrate. 'You did well guys. Make sure you drink lots of water before you go. I don't want you passing out driving home.' I congratulate the class and they give a short clap and drag back their mats. I walk over to Janet who is getting a dry towel from her bag. 'How about a coffee, Janet?' I suggest. 'Yeah, okay, but mine's an iced coffee!' and we share a conspiratory laugh.

Bronwyn is in her mid fifties and still a fitness teacher. HRT Premia 5 has reduced her body pain from severe to very mild, often she has no pain at all. Her mind is alert again and she is not anxious any more. She still has mild insomnia, usually now caused by cramps in her legs at night and having to get out of bed to go to the toilet more frequently. She takes calcium, glucosamine, a multi vitamin and an antioxidant daily. She advises young women to talk to their mothers about menopause. Bronwyn wishes she had done this before her mother passed away. She also recommends that women keep a record of dates when symptoms occur, change and cease, and a note of what is prescribed or taken. It can be difficult to remember all this information when being asked by a doctor – or a writer!

FOUR WOMEN OF A CERTAIN AGE AND MENOPAUSAL STATUS DISCUSS MATTERS OF THE UTMOST IMPORTANCE OVER LUNCH

What amazes is not that our conversation
is peppered with thingys, thingamejigs,
whatshisnames, whoziwhatsits and whatyoumacallits
but that we all know who we're talking about,
the compromising position they were in at the time,
with whom, and the names of all those implicated.
And we'd tell you too – every detail,
right down to the size and shape of their thingamabobs –
if only our blankety-blank, dooverlackie memories
        weren't so . . .
you know . . . what's that word? Bad.

Louise Nicholas

ANDREA'S STORY

Andrea's husband died eleven years ago in a car accident, leaving her with two children to raise. She is a computer analyst and was in her mid to late forties when she thought about menopause. Her periods had always been irregular so when she missed a month it was not unusual. But many of her friends were menopausal so she gathered some pamphlets and spoke to her doctor, a family member. As far as she could tell, she had no symptoms, but when she read the risk factors of osteoporosis she made an appointment to have the density of her bones tested. The results were poor.

I feel I've come to crossroads. As a younger person driving on the road of Life, I went down dirt tracks, around blind corners and into dead ends. Now, as a much older person with lots of experience behind me, I still need to improve my skills. I need to choose wisely the road I travel along for tomorrow's journey.

That's what I wrote in my journal when I turned fifty. It was strange turning fifty. Disbelief and a little fear. How is one meant to feel? I still felt young at heart, still had mountains to climb. I have a list of all the things I want to do before I pass out of this earthly life, and not many of them have been crossed off. I think life is made up of a jigsaw of decades: a decade of childhood (oh so short), a decade of adolescence (probably just as well it wasn't any longer, I might not be here now to write this story), the decade of young adulthood, my thirties, and so forth. The end of each decade challenges the beginning of a new one.

Challenge: confront, deal with, face up to, defy. I think the main reason why menopause differs from other life challenges is the matter of aging. Aging in relation to health issues and vanity issues. We arrive at a certain age and our bones start to ache, our cholesterol and blood pressure rise a little, our fitness isn't what it used to be and we put on a few kilos. We try not to think about breast cancer or heart attack and we check all the sunspots on our hands and face for any ominous changes.

I have watched my parents age. Defiance at first, playing tennis with the right elbow strapped and an elastic bandage around the left thigh from too many hamstring pulls. Muscles tearing, joints swelling and stiff. Years of physio. One day I said to them, 'Do you think you should look into playing a different sport, one that isn't too demanding on your body?' It was like a slap in the face.

You can't defy menopause. There's a lot of information to persuade a woman to go onto HRT. It supplies your body with that most valuable hormone – oestrogen. Oestrogen that helps to keep skin looking younger, longer. Tempting. I imagined the compliment: 'You're not fifty-five! You don't look a day over fifty.' Big deal! Let's face it, by the time you are menopausal, you are living in a middle-aged body looking at the world from a middle-aged face. Neither HRT, nor anything else is going to make me look ten years younger. And what happens to the youthful look when I do come off HRT? Will I be happy to age then? Of course not. So, what to do? I smear on sunscreen, wear a hat, visit my dentist regularly, smile and try to keep happy. I am often tempted to buy the miracle creams. Have you read the claims lately? Age-defying, anti-wrinkle, resilience-lifting, radiance-boosting, skin-quenching, skin-renewing, de-stressing, gravity-defying! There are creams that increase skin moisture by 76.9 per cent in six hours! Is that good enough? I ask myself. No, not when there is another cream that assists skin renewal by up to 282 per cent, but it takes a month. I can't wait that long. Ah, here is the jar I need – Overnight Success!

Do I need HRT for mood swings? I've always been a bit temperamental; it's part of my personality. Now that I am menopausal I don't think I am any more irritable or forgetful or tired than the next woman (or man for that matter). Anyway, I don't want to be too nice. I shouldn't be flippant here because I have a dear friend whose menopause was showing itself through wild mood swings, panic attacks and anxiety. She'd been feeling unworthy and unloved, both completely unjustified, but it was the way she was feeling. She experienced the whole gamut of psychological symptoms through her menopause. It was awful to see an accomplished woman in the prime of her life (forty-four) losing her confidence and crying pathetically. She had to scale down her export business for some months while she tried natural therapies supported by professional counselling and wonderful understanding from her family and friends. But after about five months of not getting the results she needed she began HRT. It took a long period of trial and error to get it right but eventually she became her self again and went back to managing her business. She's been on HRT for seven years now and is quite terrified of coming off. I mentioned this book to her and thought she had a valuable contribution to make because of her experiences. She said that the book is a wonderful idea but that she couldn't go back to that time again. She felt it would be like ripping open a deep wound.

I am lucky not to suffer from hot flushes. I haven't had one, although I do occasionally get hot in bed during the warmer weather. All my friends fan themselves over lunch, wipe their face with a serviette, go red to their hair roots, and apologise for the wet patches under their armpits. Sitting with them I am the odd one out, cool and bone dry.

I look at the list of menopause symptoms and cross off hot flushes, mood swings (there's a multitude of sub-symptoms under this heading), hair and skin changes and come to another heading – osteoporosis. That's a different matter. It's a serious disease. Thinning bones, shrinking, fractured ankles, hips, wrists. Menopause and a fall can spell disaster. I know that oestrogen is important in maintaining bone density. I can cope looking sixty when I am sixty, but I don't want to be frail with brittle bones. Am I at risk? There doesn't appear to be a family history – arthritis, yes, but that's not osteoporosis. Risk factor number one: I'm a smoker, got hooked as a teenager and tried everything to quit, and I *have* cut down drastically, but I do sneak in a smoke or two each day.

My exercise routine is sporadic. A bit of gardening isn't enough and walking Henry around the block every night isn't going to save me. I need to do some weight-bearing exercises, the pamphlet says. Risk factor number two, because I know I'll never do that.

Is my calcium intake adequate? I love cheese and chocolate, I do eat my veggies but I also wash down dinner with two or three glasses of wine. I think that's risk factor number three. A history of unreliable periods, heavy bleeding, pain reliever every month for chronic cramps – oh dear, I think I am at risk for osteoporosis.

My brother-in-law is my doctor and he referred me to have a bone-density scan. It showed levels way below average. He advised immediate oestrogen replacement therapy to prevent further bone loss and wrote out a life plan for me.

'What's it to be, Andrea? Painful osteoporosis or throw away the fags?' he said.

'I've given up,' I said not very convincingly.

'You need to exercise, too. Join a gym or club and have a proper program written out for you,' was his next suggestion. 'And I'm going to send you to a nutritionist. You need to eat a high calcium diet.'

'I eat cheese,' I retorted.

'Melted cheese on pizza doesn't count.'

Osteoporosis is the reason why I am on HRT and I made other life changes. I had therapy for my smoking and everyone was instructed to throw away any cigarettes they found. They were also allowed to be horrid to me if they smelt smoke in my hair and on my clothes. I looked into the activities that I might enjoy and persist with, and chose dancing. For the first three weeks I was so stiff and sore it was difficult to get in and out of the car and to bend down to collect Henry's offering. But it wasn't long before I was putting together a few steps and I started to feel fantastic. I have better flexibility and my legs are stronger – I no longer gasp after ten minutes. I am also feeling very proud of myself and look forward to the lessons which I attend three times a week. I am following my special diet to increase my calcium which includes soy products, fish (particularly salmon and sardines) three times a week, low-fat dairy foods, and broccoli must be on my dinner plate most nights. Snacks include almonds and dried figs and I'm allowed one glorious glass of wine a day.

I am not sure how long I will need to be on HRT. The bone-density scans will determine that. Exercising, my new life-long diet and cutting out smoking are all having a major effect on my energy and fitness, and I hope on my bones. I'm more enthusiastic about getting out there and doing things. I may even be less irritable, but I'm not sure if everyone would agree on that.

Andrea has been on HRT for three years. She recently had a bone-density scan and it showed that there had been a slight improvement. She was pleased that the treatment and her life-style changes have stopped further bone loss and, in fact, are gradually increasing the density of her bones. Sadly, her elder brother has osteoporosis. It was diagnosed after he fractured his hip from slipping on a rug.

Andrea is planning a trip to China in ten months and she is in training for climbing the hundreds of steps to the Great Wall of China. She said, 'It's the first of several things I can cross off my "want to do" list.'

DALE'S STORY

Dale's story starts when she is at university, a mature-aged student fulfilling a childhood dream of studying science. It was at this time that she started to experience confusion and difficulty in concentrating and her head ached with pressure, feelings quite foreign to Dale. She did not associate them with the onset of menopause. A year earlier her marriage had ended and she wondered if these symptoms were related to the stress of divorce.

I walked from the lecture theatre in a daze; the whiteboard, filled with equations, etched into my brain and none of it made sense. I drifted into the library and found a desk in the corner. These corrals were well sought after. There you could spread out your books and lay down your head as if you had fallen asleep studying. You were rarely disturbed. I rested my flushed cheek on the cool wood but could not nod off. My nose was blocked; my brain was stuffed.

After a rest, I stowed my books into my backpack and, leaving the hum of student activity, walked through the forest track that led to the ring road surrounding the campus. I stopped, looked along the row of abandoned cars on either side of the road and could not, for the life of me, remember where I had parked that morning. I replayed leaving home, driving to uni, getting out of the car and locking the door. I turned left and began walking. Half an hour later, I found my Mazda just fifty metres from where I had begun my search. I collapsed into the driver's seat and wondered who I was trying to kid.

I had finished high school at sixteen with a commercial course in my hand. It's what Mum said girls should do. But I envied my mates staying on for another year to do science. It's what I wanted to do. I started office work the day after sitting for my junior examination. Then I married, had kids, tried part-time work, felt frustrated, and got divorced. When, aged forty-two, I told Mum I was going to uni to study environmental science she said, 'Well dear, at least you would have tried.' Fighting words! The first few weeks at uni were great. My mind was tantalised by intriguing tasks, research and the satisfaction of finding answers.

Then came week four. It turned serious. I coped well with biology, genetics, geomorphology, climatology, even physics, but when the chemistry lecturer started speaking in formulae tongues, I lost it. For the next week, I lived in a haze. My head felt stuffed with cotton wool and I could not focus on any subject. I floundered, lost in the middle of newspaper headlines, no matter how many times I started again from the beginning. Twelve months before, when I had left my matrimonial nest of twenty years, I had braved my way through the sort of stress that only those who have been there would understand. I wondered if I was now suffering the effects of trying to hold it all together. Was I having a breakdown?

Dinners became Vegemite sandwiches. I didn't see the dust accumulating in the corners, and my embarrassing lifelong habit of spoonerising grew more acute: I told a friend I wasn't going to be 'fried till payday'. And to make matters worse, I still had a blocked nose and a temperature. Was I coming down with something? I decided to give uni one more month.

A new relationship, formed a few months before, was in that fragile, tender stage. We each bought a mountain bike. This was a big thing for me as I had never ridden a bike. I wobbled around the block, fell off, got back on and learnt how to change the gears. Weekends were precious and we went for long rides along the Brisbane River or through the bush. I liked the slow speed of this new man in my life. I did not tell him of my self-doubts.

The second month at uni proved no clearer than the first. My mind had absorbed all it could hold and each lecture and tutorial passed in a blur. I often left midway through a session, close to tears, to curl up in a corner where I could release the vice that gripped my head.

Walking through Toohey Forest one weekend, trying to identify trees using my newly acquired dichotomous key, I confessed to Doug that I was having trouble holding ideas and information in my head.

'Sometimes I think I'm going mad,' I said nervously. 'I don't think I have what it takes to be a uni student.' I removed my jumper and fanned my face with my hat. 'Not having hot flushes, are you?' Doug enquired.

'Of course not!' I retorted. Old women have hot flushes. I was only forty-two years young and in a new relationship. How dare he insult me!

That night I lay in my own bed and thought about what Doug had said. Could he be right? Soon after my third child was born, I'd had a partial hysterectomy.

Although I no longer menstruated, my life had progressed normally and I thought my hormones were in balance. For most women menopause is signalled by their change of cycle. I no longer possessed this warning device.

I took myself off to the uni medical centre. The doctor said yes, in all probability, menopause was the cause of my symptoms. He took tests and gave me a week's worth of HRT to try in the meantime to see if it made a difference. Having taken a pill immediately I went to the common room to wait for the afternoon's lecture. The chair was comfortable, the room was quiet and I fell asleep. When I awoke, I noticed something very strange. I could breathe through my nose for the first time in months. Greedily, I drew fresh air in through my nostrils. Then I noticed someone had unpacked the cotton wool from my brain and the vice no longer held my head. I went to the lecture and heard every word. I could focus, I wrote down notes, I understood. I walked to the car park thinking, I might just be able to do this degree.

'Your diagnosis was correct,' I admitted to Doug that night.

'I'm not sure what's ahead, Dale, but I'll go through this thing with you,' he said, and I was glad to have his support.

Humour helped us through. Doug said I was a source of constant amusement and I was able to laugh at my own spoonerisms instead of feeling acutely embarrassed. When I returned the next week to my doctor, he reported my hormone level had dropped 'precipitously' and I should stay on HRT. I could only agree. Although the flushes stopped they hadn't been my problem. The incapacitating dullness of my brain had, and as long as I remembered to keep taking my pills, all was well.

I managed distinctions and high distinctions in my first year and, despite being a loner, made friends with a few other mature-aged students. At home, life was full of fun and new challenges. Doug taught me how to select lengths of figured timber to make musical instruments. We went camping. We made beautiful music together. I became socially and politically aware for the first time and attended rallies.

Then one day I forgot to take my pill. Because of the build-up in my body, it took a week for the effect to show. I rose from bed in the small hours of the morning, felt for my slippers in the dark and walked for the bedroom door. Except there was no door, just a very hard wall. I heard movement from the bed then remembered I was at Doug's place. It shouldn't have been a problem to find his door, or a light switch. But I was terribly confused and had to feel my way around the room with my hands on the wall to find my way back to bed.

'Did you forget to take your pill?' Doug asked over breakfast. 'You seem all muddle-headed like you used to before you started on them.'

'No, I took it last night,' I said.

I put my pill on the table every evening beside my dinner with the salt and pepper. Still perplexed, I thought back through my week. I had stayed overnight at my mother's a few days before and had forgotten to take the pill with me. I didn't think missing one would make any difference.

'Do you really think missing one day would do this to me?' I asked Doug.

'Well, I don't know, but something has happened to you, love. You do seem a bit befuddled.'

I made a concerted effort to remember to take the pill every day. And for the next three years my grades held and so did my confidence. In year three, my biology lecturer announced there was paid fieldwork for an experienced bird-watcher. Although I wasn't qualified for the work, I offered my services.

'Would you know a yellow-faced honeyeater if you saw one?' she asked.

'No,' I said, a bit put out. 'But I know how to use a pair of binoculars and a bird book.'

A month later she rang to say that I would start on Monday. I only had the weekend to practice. Doug, an experienced birdo, took me to the forest and gave me a crash course. For the next four weeks, we rose before dawn every couple of days to observe and fill out the data sheets. Then I forgot to take a pill. A week later, I was following a compass setting, studying the map, when I looked up and the bush had lost definition. It had taken on sepia tones and looked the same in every direction. I had no idea which way I had been walking, what the map or the compass represented. I was alone and began to panic. I sat and cried until my sides ached and my head burst. Eventually, I wiped my swollen eyes and pulled myself together. I had to get to safety. Finally, I stumbled across a waterway. There is only one creek in Toohey Forest and I knew that if I followed it I would arrive either at uni or the edge of the forest.

To be so dependent on medication was soul-destroying for me. I had always been in control of my body; always held the belief that medical intervention was unnecessary if a proper diet and exercise regime was followed. I felt I had failed my body. Apart from birth control pills in my early twenties I had never taken regular drugs. Now, I could not function without them. I had bouts of embarrassing forgetfulness: standing in a supermarket wondering why I had entered and driving home empty-handed; forgetting which door in the public toilets led to the outside, which cupboard was hiding the mugs from me. And to add to my woes, journals were questioning the long-term effects of HRT.

I fulfilled my dream and at forty-five graduated with a Bachelor of Science in Environmental Studies. I continued to work with birds and took on tutoring and research work with scientists. It was at this stage that I felt strong enough to try and wean myself off HRT. I decided to go from two pills a day to one and three-quarters. A month later, one and a half, and so on until my last quarter tablet. The week following each reduction was fuzzy and hot flushes returned. But I coped well, supported by Doug, my work colleagues and friends.

The day after I had taken my last quarter tablet, I was walking along Tarn Shelf in Tasmania's Southern Highlands and every wild flower, every dew-draped spider's web smiled at me. I had made it. The rest of my life was now my own. Freedom!

Dale said she owes a debt to HRT and believes she would not have graduated without it. She looks after her health but her former doctor castigated her for giving up HRT. She said that Dale owed it to society to remain on HRT and not clog up the health system with brittle and weak bones. After a bone scan confirmed that Dale's bone density was above average for a twenty-five year old, she sought another doctor.

Dale and Doug live a happy and rewarding life together in the bush where they pursue their love for the environment and its inhabitants.

LEONE'S STORY

Leone lives amongst the rolling hills and vineyards of the beautiful Barossa Valley. She and her husband work for wineries and they love the activities surrounding the business of producing plump, sweet grapes and turning them into wine. Leone has two adult children and a very close family. She was forty-seven when her menopause symptoms and subsequent trials of hormone replacement therapy created chaos in her life.

I live in Freeling where the TV program *McLeod's Daughters* is filmed. There is the Gungellan Pub and the Gungellan Truck Stop in the main street and every few weeks the sleepy little town turns into a busy metropolis with film crew setting up cameras, speakers, lights and props. Freeling is surrounded by crop farmers so as well as seeing helicopters drop off actors we also see harvesters, ploughs, hay-baling, sheep and tractors. I love it here.

I'm a country girl. I spent most of my childhood in the Barossa and lived many years in Naracoorte bringing up my children. I've lived in the city, too, but I felt constantly stressed by the noise, traffic and number of people around me. However, city living gave my kids more educational and employment opportunities.

So here I am in Freeling, back in the Barossa Valley,

with my second husband, Tony. Tony and I have been married for just over three years. I was a single mum for fifteen years, worked full-time and had little respite. My kids are now young adults and have gone and come back and gone again. My daughter is currently living with us, working twelve-hour shifts on the vintage. Tony, who doesn't have children of his own, loves my kids and has a close relationship with them.

Tony places no demands on me. He's supportive, affectionate, communicative and a real character. We are both independent with strong personalities and we think differently. It's been quite an adjustment and, although we drive each other nuts at times, we have happily settled into our peaceful 100-year-old cottage with its creaking floorboards and crooked door frames. We love to sit under its bull-nose verandah, gently rocking on the swing-seat on a warm summer's night supping a cold beer. Our two dogs doze on our laps while galahs and cockatoos settle into the trees for the night and frogs and crickets compete with each other. And most summer mornings we see colourful hot air balloons floating in the sky taking lucky passengers to Seppeltsfield for a champagne breakfast.

Sound idyllic? But just as surely as a stormy winter follows a blissful summer, so too does life change. *The* change. I have been on an emotional roller-coaster for twelve months now and I'm bloody sick of it. I feel that everything about me has changed. Nothing is familiar, physically or mentally. I hate my body now. HRT has been a nightmare and I am twelve kilograms heavier. I feel ugly and fat. I've been comfort eating to make me feel better but, of course, it only makes me feel worse. When I look in a mirror I feel miserable and go and eat a chocolate or a lolly.

A year ago my life turned upside down when I went to my doctor feeling crook. I flinched in pain when he pressed over my appendix. Over the next twenty-four hours I had numerous blood tests for cancer and an ultrasound that showed a large pelvic mass. The results confirmed an ovarian cyst the size of a rock melon. I had both ovaries removed as another cyst was forming on the other ovary. Because of the size of the cyst I was cut across my abdomen and it was removed very carefully with both hands so as not to burst it. Pathology revealed a borderline ovarian cancer totally contained within the middle of the cyst.

This all happened so quickly, I was in shock. I acted normally but I was scared to death. There was the ultra-sound technician who hovered over one spot for ages and then disappeared to consult with someone else, leaving me wondering if everything was okay. And the doctor who was so blasé when he said that more tests were needed to check for cancer elsewhere in my body. That word sent shivers up and down my spine. No thought was given to my feelings. I felt like a number. The days were filled with appointments and tests and I got through them on automatic pilot. The evenings were the worst. All that time to think. Tony later admitted that he was petrified but at the time neither of us wanted to talk about it. My son cried when I told him and my daughter returned home from overseas.

I was in hospital for seven days and it took two months to recover. In Australia, one woman every ten hours is diagnosed with ovarian cancer so I am truly grateful to those who located the cyst accidentally while trying to find my appendix, and to the surgeon who carefully removed the growth. It was recommended that I consult a cancer specialist in three and six months, then annually to check that no more cysts were forming. The onset of menopause was never mentioned.

Hot flushes started about a week after the operation. They came from deep within my upper chest and radiated from the inside out and up to the very top of my head. It was instant heat and came with no warning. I broke out into a sweat and had to fan myself furiously to cool down. They would last for several minutes and I had about six to ten a day. Hot night sweats woke me several times a night. Whereas the daytime flushes were from my neck up, the night sweats covered my whole body.

I went to see an obstetrician/gynaecologist. I said that I wasn't keen to go onto HRT and would prefer to try natural products. He laughed and said that they wouldn't work and that I would be wasting my time and money. He also warned me against some natural remedies because my family has a history of cancer. My father died from cancer at fifty-two, my sister is a survivor of breast cancer and two of my grandparents died of cancer. I had also watched something on TV not long before which associated some natural products with cancer. This scared me. I trusted my specialist so shrugged my shoulders and accepted what he said to be true. I had already tried natural products for hot flushes and they hadn't worked for me, so what the doctor said made sense.

I started HRT (Estrofem) three weeks after my operation and although this stopped the hot flushes in the day, I continued to have night sweats. I immediately gained weight and suffered from several other menopausal symptoms: mood swings, insomnia, fatigue, headaches, body aches, poor memory and confusion. To help alleviate these, the specialist prescribed Livial in addition to Estrofem.

After six months I told him that although I was feeling better, I was still feeling old, confused, tired and my body ached. My breasts became painfully engorged and my nipples were itchy. So he changed my HRT again, taking me off Estrofem and doubling the Livial.

'Is this as good as it gets?' I asked him. 'Should I just accept that I feel ten years older?'

'Certainly not!' he said. 'You're only forty-eight. That's young and feeling anything less than normal is unacceptable to me.' I left with my hopes raised. I was driving home and when I turned into our street a kangaroo was sitting in the middle of the road right in front of our cottage. Amazing! It was probably looking for water and food because of the drought. It hopped away down the streets of Freeling. I laughed to myself and thought this is what people from other countries think Australia is all about. It was a momentary relief before my symptoms worsened and I thought I was going crazy.

Tony noticed a change in my personality within days. I verbally attacked this wonderful man, feeling angry and depressed, wondering if I had made a mistake marrying him. I constantly cried and thought about running away from home. I couldn't finish a sentence as I would forget what I was saying. Crying into the phone, I made another appointment. The specialist took me off Livial and back onto Estrofem at double the original dose. He ordered blood tests to check my hormone levels and also to rule out diabetes and any thyroid problem.

'Do you think I could be depressed?' I asked.

'Yes, I think you are,' he answered. 'I can't help you there; you'll have to see your GP for a script.'

'Could I try without HRT?' I suggested.

'You can't go off it!' He seemed shocked at the idea. 'You will feel like an old woman.'

'But I feel like one now,' I cried.

'It's not an option. Your hot flushes will return and drive you mad.' He dismissed me.

My gynaecologist seemed to be only concerned with the flushes that had disappeared a few days after I started HRT. But to me, the flushes were the least of my worries. When I mentioned my body aches, sore breasts, memory loss, fatigue and, recently, cramps in my legs, he all but ignored me. I was his last appointment for the day and he really couldn't be bothered. He was a nice guy and a good doctor, but he just didn't get it! The blood test results showed my hormones to be normal and *he* was satisfied. He'd done his job. As long as the numbers were correct, it seemed that how *I* was feeling was irrelevant. I left in tears, confused, rejected and with boobs ready to burst. If I had a smidgen of confidence left in me, it evaporated.

The GP gave me antidepressants without batting an eyelid. Nothing else was suggested. I've thought about seeing another specialist but my experience has left me doubting if any male can possibly understand or relate to menopause. It's on my list to see a female specialist. There has to be a better solution.

Sitting in my swing-seat I can hear the CFS siren being tested. It's Thursday evening training and I say a quiet thank you to those fantastic volunteers who work hard to keep us safe from bush fires. I'm stuffing myself with chocolates, feeling fat and ugly. Tony joins me, lays a hand on mine and asks how I am. I snap an answer feeling irritable. He cares for me so well and I'm trying hard to like my husband again. My next visit to the specialist is a month away. He has suggested an oestrogen implant, but I'm unsure. I'm searching for answers and solutions because I just want to be *me* again. Although I am feeling better – not great, just okay, just getting through each day on little sleep – there is still so much to contend with. My knees hurt, my ankles hurt and even my toes hurt. I have to be careful with my back when I bend. My hips are sore and I cannot lie on my side for longer than ten minutes, so I toss and turn all night to relieve my aches and pains. I get headaches and my neck and shoulders feel stiff. Perhaps it's arthritis; I do have arthritis in my thumbs. Perhaps it's the extra weight I'm carrying; I must do something about that. Perhaps it's nearing fifty years old; my doctor says that's still young. Perhaps I should accept how I'm feeling. No! My specialist is happy with HRT; I'm not.

Because of the operation and all the associated worry over cancer, then the hormonal aftermath and the trials and errors of HRT, I have lost my confidence. I've been a single mother for goodness sake! There have been many hurdles and upheavals, and I've made all sorts of decisions concerning myself and my kids. So why can't I handle a simple thing like menopause?

I must take control of my life. I must make wise choices.

I decided to have the oestrogen implant which was placed under the skin where my right ovary used to be. The specialist said that the oestrogen should last between six and twelve months, and that hot flushes would indicate that the implant was empty. Immediately my breasts became engorged and painful with very itchy nipples. I had to hold my breath when I removed my bra and a hug was out of the question. It was over three months before the pain eased and I had about two months of some normality. Then in the sixth month of the implant my menopause symptoms returned. I felt teary, tired and sore everywhere. I became intolerant and muddled again, my moods swinging wildly. And this is my current state. I have no hot flushes but if these symptoms do not settle down soon, I will need to see my specialist again.

I have joined a gym for the first time in my life and go three times a week. I reckon that is as good a therapy as any at the moment. I'm enjoying it and want to lose fifteen kilograms. I tried yoga but it wasn't for me. I am hoping that once I have lost some weight and I'm feeling healthier and fitter, that my whole 'self' will return. I just want to be *me* again.

Leone is still searching for a solution to her menopause. She has the name of an alternative practitioner who specialises in 'Reconnective Healing'. The brochure states that this is a natural therapy which works with the energy centres of the body to raise levels of wellbeing and self-confidence. There are no drugs, so she has nothing to lose and everything to gain.

PAULA'S STORY

Paula is a sole parent with a teenage son. She manages a small team in the media, preparing deadline-based broadcast content. She follows current affairs with a passion driven by a belief that the world could be a far better place. An activist for many years, there is always a campaign she is supporting. Paula was fifty-two when she realised she was menopausal and this is the story of her first twelve months.

The shift from summer to autumn can catch you out. It's not the season for flannelette pyjamas, or the singlet and jumper. But it's no longer T-shirt weather either. There had been a run of warm weather at the beginning of autumn and in its second month I start to dress by the book. But I'm not getting it right. The PJs are unpacked but I'm far too warm to wear them; I've even flung off the blanket. And the singlet under the jersey knit is a tad warm. At work I sigh, 'I'm so tired, just not sleeping. I'm awake at two or three, then four and six.' Yawning at my workstation I carry on, feeling like a truck has hit me.

Weeks pass and I am now waking in a lather of perspiration, kicking the blankets off and pushing my limbs out to find cool air. I am burning, like a radiator switched up high. A few minutes later it's as if the switch is turned off and I need the blanket back. This goes on all through the night; a blur of half doze.

Then it dawns on me. Oh no! This is it. Menopause. The end. I hate the word. There's defeat and a level of social shame. It's common knowledge that menopause marks the time when you start to go loopy. You can't be trusted to make decisions and you become erratic. Colour drains from your hair and skin loses its elasticity. Bones ache, your fanny dries up – STOP!

Forget any of the big O's. The fortieth birthday party was just that – a party! The fiftieth was a hoot. I have had just two years' grace and I am menopausal. I quietly nurse the knowledge that I have entered this stage of life. I wish I could ask some questions because I need answers urgently. Will it get worse? For how long will it go on? What are the treatments? But embarrassment holds me back. No one talks about menopause! I start to look at my friends in a new way wondering who has beaten me to the line. Could I broach the subject? It would mean making the assumption – the accusation – that they are menopausal. But I'm desperate. I casually bring it into conversation. Clearly it's an illness.

'Have you seen a doctor?' they ask. 'Don't muck around, get onto HRT,' they counsel. I take their advice and see a doctor. She asks about symptoms. I talk in an offhand manner about flushes and insomnia, anxiety and moodiness. (I don't mention the bristles on my chin and scaly skin appearing on the back of my upper arms. They are too much to admit.) She is older than I am and nods knowingly. Do I detect smugness? Is that a certain glow of victory in her encouraging smile? I pull myself together and ask her if it will get worse and for how long I must endure this hell.

'There are no answers, every woman is different,' she says. 'A woman will have her own combination of symptoms and the severity with which they strike. Some women detect changes that vanish in months. Others might suffer for ten years. There's no telling which way it will go for you at this stage.'

This is not what I want to hear. She advises me to walk and attend to relaxation, to take a cup of hot milk at bedtime, to tuck into soya products and pulses. An appointment is suggested in a few months' time when my patterns might be clearer. There is no mention of HRT and I'm relieved not to embark on a life of medication ... after all, how would you know when to stop? I leave dissatisfied and depressed, doomed to a purgatory of waiting.

Months have passed without a period. I am reminded of a feminist slogan: Biology is not destiny. Who the hell came up with that? Biology was on my mind each month for those two crippling days leading into my period. I carried a dull backache and overwhelming fatigue. And biology is on my mind again, now that I am finding my way through menopause. I don't miss my periods. There's a level of comfort in being amongst the 'average' group of women whose bleeding stops between fifty and fifty-one. I have crossed sanitary pads off the shopping list and replaced them with panty liners. I wonder when I'll have to upsize to incontinence pads? Things are changing. I catch myself absentmindedly pulling at a wayward bristle on the chin, and remind myself not to do this in public.

Last week I was riding my bicycle home through the city. I passed younger women strolling in those silly hipster pants, their muffin top exposed and flaunted. They think they are young forever. I rode on and passed a picket line of stalwarts with their placards calling for motorists to toot for rights for refugees. I rang my bell as I pulled up at the lights. Then an elderly woman waved and started to come towards me. Who could it be? It took me ages to realise it was a friend of many years whom I'd not seen for eighteen months. We'd had our boys at the same time and had stayed friends through their growing up.

'Pat,' I exclaimed and scooted to the footpath, hoping she had not noticed my failure to recognise her. 'How are you?' I gushed, appalled at the lines on her face, her thinning grey hair and her physical transformation into a brick. We exchanged bits of news, said our goodbyes and promised to catch up soon. I pedalled on my way and caught sight of my reflection in the shop windows. An aged woman stared back at me. She too was a brick. Another of life's horror-filled revelations. It's not fair. I still feel twenty, wild and reckless. I still ride my bike without a light, and sneak through red lights and scream abuse at motorists who cut me off. I still roll out of bed, pick my clothes up from the floor, shower and dress and head to work inside half an hour. Hell, I still do cartwheels!

I was in my mid thirties when I first noticed I was gaining weight. I was lolling in an armchair, idly pinching my stomach and realised I had a 'spare tyre'. It was more a racing bike tyre than the Mack truck tube I hoist along with me these days. Back then I marvelled at the arrival of what I called 'the alien'. Now I pat the rolls with the familiarity you'd offer the family pet. I have observed my own transformation with some dismay. I caught myself the other day descending into the armchair with an unrepressed grunt!

Biology is reality. How is a woman expected to perform (and be happy) when struck down every month by menstruation and its debilitating symptoms? There are no less than twenty-four 'common' symptoms in the brochures. And just when her periods stop, finally, after about thirty-five years, she starts the next stage of her life – menopause. There's a great choice of symptoms here; it's too scary even to mention them. Biology is on my mind again now that I am finding my way through insomnia, anxiety, sweats and depression. Biology is reality. Women's experiences are different. The bonus of this mammoth endurance is, apparently, that we live longer! I can add grumpy, short-tempered and rude to being constantly tired. The fuse is short these days. My tolerance is limited. I rub everyone up the wrong way at work (I've bitten only one person's head off this week). I'm amused by the half-baked ideas of the young.

It's time to say what I think, time for a bit of telling it like it is. No longer will I be a doormat for the sake of keeping the peace, protecting other people's feelings. What about my feelings? I have a new confidence, backed up by a wealth of insight and experience but the new What about me? is getting me into trouble – nobody likes being caught out by the Bullshit Detector.

I have joined a witches' coven and twice a day go through the ritual of taking the Black Cohosh. There are nuts and seeds to chew and quotas of soy products to ingest. The meat sacrifices are becoming larger. Fruit pieces are laid out in lines. Sugar is the devil's food and is banned. And I drink buckets of pure water hourly. The coven hangs around in gangs and went to the movies last week. We trooped into the Ladies before the film. We trooped in again when it finished. We found a café and ordered hot chocolate. We screeched with laughter at the nonsense we'd just seen and the word 'incontinence' was uttered.

Barb, suddenly serious, confided, 'I can't run anymore.' 'No,' chimed in another, 'can't laugh either.' Dancing's a risk and there's certainly no jumping for joy!

The body, showing signs of decrepitude, must be attended to. I am noticing an ache in the hip, a general stiffness, and a pinched sciatica which can shoot a pain through me that stops me in my tracks. The process must be stalled. So I join circles of women in darkened rooms where we lie on the floor and roll and stretch and conclude chanting our om's, seeking peace. This is the closest thing to deep sleep I get.

Paula says she is plotting a way out of the relentless and exhausting work in the media and is hatching a plan to go part-time. Sharing a community garden-plot fulfills her love of gardening, and nature walks in the bush give her a degree of emotional restoration and she enjoys reading, writing and films.

She has managed her menopause using Remifem and herbals, a diet high in phytoestrogens, exercise and relaxation techniques.

STEPHANIE'S STORY

Stephanie was forty-seven when perimenopause started. She was married with two adult sons living at home accompanied by their girlfriends on regular occasions. Although she worked for a large medical centre and had doctors and pamphlets on menopause available to her, she still felt awkward and confused.

After laying my book on the bedside table at ten, I switch off the lamp and close my red eyes. I practise emptying my head of all thoughts, I take long, slow breaths and I relax every muscle in my body. Just past midnight and I am still awake. Greg is snoring next to me and a chorus of snores comes from the boys' bedrooms. A night sweat comes quickly, sticking to my legs. I can feel the sweat trickling behind my knees and pooling in my groin. The quilt is thrown aside and I dangle my legs out. The cool air on my feet gives instant relief. I press the flannelette PJs to my legs and soak up the sweat. I'm shivering now. I swing my legs back onto the bed and pull the quilt over. Brrr. I curl into a ball and try to get warm again but my legs are clammy from the damp PJs. I quietly get out of bed and go to the bathroom to wipe my legs properly with a flannel and towel. I sprinkle talcum powder liberally from my waist down and put on another pair of PJs. I creep back to bed and start all over again. Deep, slow breathing. Relax. Keep calm. Greg's snores reach full volume. And I lay fretting now because it's 2.30 am and I am still awake. I am trying too hard to relax and can feel my stomach knotting up. Dawn is breaking and I hear the first chirps from birds. Tears seep from my eyes and roll down into my ears. And then I sleep.

'Morning,' I greet Greg. My sons are still in bed. Still snoring.

'Oh, good morning,' says Greg, looking at the clock. 'Alright for some to sleep in. I had a bloody awful night. Turn your electric blanket off. The sheets were bloody wringing wet.'

'Sorry. It's not the blanket, I don't have it on. I think I've started menopause.'

Greg stares blankly for a second, then walks away saying, 'What's that gonna mean?'

'Don't really know much about it. I still have periods although they're not normal. I missed last month's.'

'You're not pregnant?' Greg asks, suddenly alarmed.

'No, I think it's all to do with menopause. I'm getting hot flushes too.'

But Greg is not listening and the back door slams shut behind him. He's gone to clean his car. He doesn't do it himself, he takes it to a car wash every Saturday morning. He starts the car, winds down the window and shouts to me, 'Make sure the boys are ready by eleven.' And the throb of his V8 disappears down the driveway. He'll be back in time to pick the boys up for footy.

I put the kettle on, drop two pieces of bread into the toaster and walk into the laundry to put the washing machine on. The boys stay in bed and crawl out with ten minutes to get ready. I pack sandwiches, fruit cake and make two flasks of sweet coffee. They all leave with a blast from the horn and my eldest lets me know that Jeanette will be around for dinner.

I pick up, put away, change the bed sheets, hang out the washing, feed the dog, pull a few weeds and cook. I put my feet up with a cuppa just before I hear the car roar up the driveway. They're miserable. Geelong lost. Jeanette and I pretend we care. We set the table and eat the egg and bacon pie I have made. It's their favourite meal after football. After I clear the table and wash the dishes we all sit around the telly to watch the evening match. Then I go to bed with my book. And the night sweats start again.

That is how my menopause began. My periods became less frequent and then would come back with a vengeance. The night sweats caused insomnia and the lack of sleep started to affect everything I did. I worked for a medical practice and we had some pamphlets on menopause. All the information advised HRT and I knew that the doctors within the practice would recommend the same. I was hesitant because my grandmother died of breast cancer and my mother always said not to take it. She'd managed so why couldn't I? None of my girlfriends mentioned anything about menopause although we were all similar in age.

One evening after footy, we went with friends to a Thai restaurant and halfway through the spicy food I thought I was going to die. Hot flushes were setting me on fire, my clothes were clinging to my body and sweat was pouring off my face into my dinner. I went to the bathroom where I stripped to my underwear, not caring who came in. I washed myself with the paper towels provided and dried my top under the hand-blower. Greg was furious with me that night, said that he had never been so embarrassed. I had

noticed this burning-up effect before when I had cooked a curry.
Wine, too, had the same horrible effect. So I cut out hot spicy food
and alcohol.

I arrive for work a few minutes late. The reception
area is full of impatient patients. The phone is ringing and
I answer. My mind is completely blank for a few seconds.
What's the name of the centre? I give my name instead and
ask how I may help. It works. A doctor asks for his next
patient's file and I am confused. We have an excellent
system of files, special pigeon holes, colour coded—a system
that I established and have used for four years. But I can't
think straight and I try to cover up my panic by sounding
super efficient. I can feel the heat rising to my hair roots
and lately I notice that my heart races when I feel this
way. I now think I have a heart condition. I skip my breaks
and lunches because I am so behind in my work.

I begin to dread work. I can't rely on myself and my
self-esteem is all but shattered. I don't think anyone has
noticed my state, no one has said anything to me. We are all
so busy at work and I admit that I do not show much care
for other colleagues either. Someone might say that she has
a sore throat and the only sympathy she gets is, 'Well keep
away from me, I don't want it.' I feel a wreck and after an
anxious time when I mix up some blood samples I make an
appointment to see one of the doctors.

'I think I need a general checkup, haven't had one for a
few years and I'm feeling a bit run down,' I say casually.
I don't want to admit that I feel like a crazy woman.
I don't want to lose my job. He takes my blood pressure,
takes a blood sample and all the while chats warmly to
me. He asks me to describe my run-down bits. He's
so nice, I start to cry. I feel like a kid and want my mum to

hug me. Somehow I let slip about my racing heart because I'm really worried about it.

'How long have you been feeling like this?' he asks as I button up my blouse after he's done a pap smear and breast and pelvic examination.

'Oh, I guess a couple of years. It's a bit hard to tell, but I have been feeling worse these last six months.' He asks me more questions and I'm feeling stupid and embarrassed because I'm trying so hard to follow what he is saying. I mumble something about my periods being irregular and not sleeping, and while he's writing all this down I break out into an almighty hot flush, drenching my blouse.

'You're menopausal, Stephanie. Do you know that?' he says looking over his reading glasses.

'Oh yes, of course I do,' I answer not wanting to appear a complete idiot.

'Then it's HRT for you my girl and all your troubles will vanish.'

In some ways this sounds so comforting, so simple and easy. But I think of my grandmother and mention this to him in a professional manner.

'Taking HRT doesn't mean you will get breast cancer.' He goes on to explain the benefits including the protective effect on my heart and saying that without hormone therapy I am at risk of osteoporosis, 'Which is very serious, Stephanie.' He explains the prescription, saying that he wants to see me again in a fortnight. I am dismissed and feel that my consultation is rushed.

I leave feeling dissatisfied but don't know what else I can do. I go to the chemist, hand over my prescription, and take home a packet of pills. The relief is almost immediate. I feel human again. The night sweats and hot flushes during the day almost disappear and I can sleep. Glorious sleep. A fortnight passes and I see my doctor again.

'You see, I told you HRT would fix your problems,' he proudly says. He knows he is right. I ask how long I will need to be on the pills.

'Forever! Why would you want to come off them?' But he corrects himself when he sees my astonished face and says, for a while, reminding me that when I do stop the menopause symptoms will reappear. He says to continue and come and see him if I have any concerns.

Greg is thrilled to have his old Steph back. A happy wife with energy to clean the house, cook the meals and willing to have sex. I am efficient at work, forget nothing, and can't believe the amount of spare time I have on my hands. My periods return to normal, no more unexpected flooding. But there is a little niggle in the back of my brain which I choose to ignore for the present time.

I stayed on HRT for a year and then decided to try and come off it. The hot flushes and night sweats returned accompanied by sleepless nights, and I almost ran to the chemist for another prescription. While I was taking HRT my life was as it always had been but I knew I would eventually have to come off the pills, regardless of what my doctor said. I stopped five years later. I was fifty-five. My periods quickly became very light and infrequent, stopping within four months. I had no hot flushes during the day and although the night sweats returned, they were infrequent and mild. But other symptoms appeared or reappeared. My libido had drained from me long ago and whether on HRT or not it didn't come back. I don't think I can blame menopause for the loss of my libido. When I was young, very young, I was just as keen as Greg. Then

I gave birth to my sons and my libido was on and off for years depending on my tiredness and the worries for their happiness and their future. But menopause was to blame for a dry vagina, sometimes making intercourse very painful for me. It frustrated Greg very much. He has always been what I would call a vigorous lover, although I don't think there was much love. I was the outlet for his sexual desires. It was always about how long he could hold on, his stamina. He saw it as a challenge, trying for everlasting youth. But changes do happen and couples need to understand and accept. When I asked him to be more gentle, he was very put out. Neither of us fully understood the implications of menopause and sexuality. In any case, I don't think it would have made a difference; sex had become an obligation for me and Greg wasn't prepared to adjust.

I do not regret those early menopausal years. I had been married for twenty-seven years when the first signs appeared and my life quickly became chaotic. As a wife and mother, daughter and sister, employee and friend, I had always been reliable, organised and caring. Those two years trying to work and cope were frightening for me. It was a very lonely and confusing time. And it was a time when I really needed understanding, love and support. I didn't get it. I know this was partly my fault but no one talked about menopause. My female colleagues and girlfriends knew very little and were embarrassed to talk about it. It was as if I had a contagious disease. Once, I tried to explain to Mum how I was feeling, but she never suffered herself and I could see that she thought I was a bit crazy. Which I was. She made me chicken broth and said, 'Now get that into you. You'll feel a lot better.' She also said that I ought to get Greg and the boys to help more. I knew this.

When I went onto HRT I saw my life clearly. Of course it wasn't really the HRT itself, it was having gone through that ghastly time and my family leaving me to get on with it. I needed help, physical help with the chores and emotional support. I got neither. And it wasn't that Greg and my sons didn't realise this; it was obvious. Greg had to remind me to make the beds when I had forgotten; the fridge was regularly bare of essentials like bread, fruit and cheese. Once, I brought the washing in off the line and threw it all back in the washing machine thinking it was a basket of dirty clothes. I cried a lot and Greg and my boys turned away, not knowing how to help, or even trying. It was only after looking back on that time that I made an important decision. I left. Of course there were other factors but my suffering from menopause and being left to handle it on my own was the straw that broke the camel's back (or rather mine!). When I put my suitcase into the boot of my car, Greg came rushing out the back door and shouted, 'After all I've gone through.' The next couple of years were not easy, but that's another story.

Stephanie is now fifty-eight years old. Just prior to taking her last HRT pill she sought advice from alternative health practitioners and, after talking to several, selected a female naturopath. Although Stephanie is post the pause she knows she must care for her body taking heed of her old doctor's warning about osteoporosis. She combines calcium supplements with a diet high in phytoestrogens, has regular medical checkups and has become quite skilled in yoga and meditation. Her sons are both married, Jeanette is now her daughter-in-law and she has a granddaughter. She wishes she could be around for her granddaughter's menopause. 'But at least she has my story to read.'

BRING IT ON

Men, of course
do not bleed
or bloat
each month,
more or less,
though they may
live with one of a kind
who does.
Forty years
of regular red.
The article said
the average age
to kiss goodbye
to blood and birth
is fifty-one.
I'm overdue by
twenty-four above average
periods of not knowing
if blood marks the chair
after I'm there,
of wide-eyed nights
fire-face flushes,
touch-me-not breasts,

and metronome moods.
Menopause?
Bring it on.
And don't you bloody dare
Tell me I'm hormonal.

Robyn Lance

KAREN'S STORY

Karen had a relatively new partner when early menopause started. She feared this would threaten her relationship because they had been trying for a child.

I wasn't ready for Mother Nature to stop my child-bearing years. If I had fallen pregnant at forty-three I would have been thrilled. So would've Simon, my partner. We have a brood of four, sometimes five kids. I have two children from a previous marriage, Simon also two whom we have on a fifty-fifty share basis with their mother, and we have my father stay with us to give my mum a break from his Alzheimer's. We wanted a child together, kept trying, and were hopeful. So when my period didn't turn up one month, menopause was the furthest thing from my mind. I didn't rush off to have a pregnancy test; I have had two miscarriages and have learnt to wait for three months. When my period didn't show in the second month, I allowed a small smile to appear on my lips. But in the third month I had some spotting. I went to the doctor who told me I wasn't pregnant and that I may be perimenopausal. She might as well have told me I had cancer and had three months to live. I handled it pretty badly. I argued with her and said that I was far too young to be menopausal and that

I had no symptoms to indicate this. She knew me quite well and I felt that I could take this liberty with her.

While I was driving home, I realised that I knew virtually nothing about menopause. I had never thought about it before. I kept thinking, 'Surely that's something that happens when I'm at least fifty. I want another child!'

When I arrived home Simon had a cup of tea ready for me and asked me what Beverley had said. I couldn't tell him. Simon is seven years younger than me and I suddenly felt ancient as I stood in front of him. 'Another miscarriage,' I said and sat down. He put his arm around my shoulders and said, with a smile around his eyes, 'We'll have to keep trying.' Yes, I determined, and took a sip of my tea. I'm not menopausal!

The next two months I had two normal periods, the third month some spotting and the fourth nothing. A very light period arrived sometime in the middle of the fifth month followed by another spotting two weeks later. My periods never returned after that. I could no longer deny that I was menopausal. Other symptoms were arriving, mainly night sweats and some hot flushes during the day. Fortunately it was summer and I could get away with not telling Simon. I let things glide along and pushed menopause to the furthest corner of my mind. This was easy to do in a very busy household.

Simon and I had been together for three years when my menopause showed its ugly face. Nothing really worries Simon; he's fun loving, great with the kids, gives Dad his shower and helps him in the toilet. He loves camping and photography, he's messy like me and is the only man I know who isn't afraid to cry. To me, that means he's emotionally mature. So different from my first husband who was emotionally tight, career driven; who travelled and brought home lots of presents, but was rarely at home. Simon makes a good living from his photography in addition to his framing business. And what do I do? I hate that question. I raise my kids and run the house. I get up and shower at seven in the morning and sink into bed around midnight and sometime between those hours I do book-keeping for three clients who have small businesses.

Simon and I had kept nothing from each other. We'd talked about our pasts, our faults and regrets, and promised to be open. And there I was, keeping the biggest secret from him. During those six months when my periods were on and off I would not acknowledge menopause. I forced myself not to think about it. But when my periods stopped and I started to feel very menopausal I realised that I had to tell Simon. I felt burdened and sick, especially when we made quiet love in the evenings and he whispered, 'Perhaps this month.' And because I was holding out on him, I had to grieve the end of my menses on my own. I felt the loss deeply. No more babies, never again, ever. As well as trying to cope with this reality was the fear that I could lose Simon. I had been in a relationship for three years with a much younger man who wanted another child and I just couldn't accept that I was menopausal. I really thought that I was far too young to be at that stage of my life.

Being menopausal and fearful is not a good mix. I became anxious and unsure of myself. The night sweats and anxiety kept me awake at night and days became a confused blur. I could not afford to be tired and pushed myself to do my normal day's work. It wasn't long before I was forgetting things, explainable things at first. I forgot to pick up the girls from tennis practice; they had tried to phone me but I was at the shops with my mobile phone off. It wasn't until I returned home and unloaded the boot with groceries and walked into a quiet house, that I realised the girls had been waiting for me for over an hour. I had never forgotten them before. One day I was doing a client's MYOB and I couldn't do it. Work I had done a hundred times and I couldn't think, couldn't focus and couldn't remember. I put my head in my hands and thought, 'What the hell is happening to me?' This only made me more anxious and I started to doubt if anyone could trust me. Could I trust myself?

It was Simon who broached the subject, one Sunday evening. We were alone. He cooked chicken with pickled lemons and wild rice for dinner, my favourite. We shared a bottle of white wine and moved to the lounge suite.

'You've started menopause, haven't you?' Although he was holding my hand and said it gently, I felt like he had slapped me. I felt so guilty and mumbled some apology. 'There's no need to apologise for being menopausal, but you do need to apologise for not telling me,' he said, still holding my hand. 'It wasn't difficult to put missed periods and hot flushes together and come up with menopause. I was waiting for you to tell me in your own time. But when you didn't and when I noticed that you were suffering in other ways, I had to get it out in the open.'

I sat very still, unable to talk, waiting for the bombshell. It never came. Simon talked to me for what seemed like hours. 'We have four lovely kids ... more than most ... we're so lucky ... we have each other ... we have so much to look forward to ...' He was talking about a future, together, and I shook with relief.

Over the next few days and nights we talked at length

about the symptoms that I was experiencing and what menopause would mean to both of us. Simon quickly came to terms with not having another child. He reasoned, 'We've been trying for two years, had two miscarriages, and I was already quite prepared for the fact that it wasn't likely to happen.' I took longer, but as my body succumbed to menopause the tension of wishing for and wanting another child gradually diminished.

I was in my second year of menopause when I visited Dr Beverley again. The flushes and night sweats disturbed my sleep and I was constantly tired. I had regular headaches which I think may have been caused by the effort of not forgetting anything. And I was anxious over every small thing. Simon was treating my menopause like a school project and researched everything. Over the dinner table he read out the latest bit of information he had downloaded. 'I don't want to know,' I bit back. I was still in denial but that's when I acknowledged that I needed some help.

'What do you think you need help with the most?' asked Bev.

'Something for the flushes so that I can sleep, and I just want to feel alive again,' I sighed. Bev said that HRT is very effective for my symptoms, particularly flushes, but I hesitated. My mother's sister had breast cancer in her early fifties and my mother has had a history of thrombosis. I thought that these two factors, so close to home, constituted an unnecessary risk. I asked about alternatives and we discussed some self-care measures I could do. I wanted to try these in the first place, the safest things, and if they didn't work then I would try the next safest.

For the flushes I cut out all spicy food. I also reduced alcohol to one glass of cold white wine two or three times a week. I found that red wine would bring on a flush. I cut down on hot beverages such as soups and coffee and made, instead, cold milk drinks with dollops of yoghurt. This had the added benefit of boosting my calcium intake. I made cold soups and found them delicious, especially fresh tomato and basil or cucumber and mint. Because we live in Queensland, cutting down on hot drinks was easier to do than if living in a cold climate. I wore pure cotton clothes and tied up my hair. It's amazing how hot I became with my hair hugging my neck and so piling it up was an easy and effective way of keeping cooler. In addition, I increased my water to six glasses a day. I found this quite difficult for a couple of weeks until a friend suggested I carry a drink with me everywhere – in the car, in my shopping bag – and on the first day I drank bottles of water without realising it.

I didn't need to change my diet very much because I eat a lot of fruit and vegetables every day. I did change from white bread to wholemeal, or soy and linseed, and increased my intake of soy products. I found the best way was drink more soy milk drinks and I take a high potency soy supplement which also includes calcium, magnesium and vitamin D3.

I am always on the go and when exercises were suggested I wondered how I would have the energy or the time. I decided that what I needed were relaxation exercises, so Simon and I joined a yoga group. Initially we all met in a park with our mats, but I found the outside weather too humid. Instead of relaxing, I was swatting insects away from my face and getting hot and frustrated. So we bought a yoga DVD and unwound in our own home with the curtains closed and muted music. Very effective. When we got bored with the same DVD and exercises, we bought another one of a different type of yoga and we now have a selection including Pilates. I have found stretching wonderful just before going to bed and again in the morning. It releases my tension and has helped to control my headaches. Massage, too, has been very beneficial, improving my circulation and relaxing my muscles. Although Simon is willing and does a great job, I try to have a professional massage once a month. I think the time of day is very important for massage. I have had a massage in the morning, only to do shopping on the way home and clean and cook for a couple of hours. By the end of the day I feel that I have lost the benefits of the massage. I prefer to time my massage when all the day's chores are done and I have nothing else to do but enjoy the massage, relax and sleep.

These practices have helped me cope better with my menopause. My flushes haven't gone but they are bearable and I wake less during the night. I'm not a Duracel battery but I have a little more energy during the day, and because I sleep better I can get through the day without too many dramas. As long as I drink plenty of water, have rest and exercise, my headaches keep away. As you can see, I'm not on top of the world but I do not feel that I need medication.

I read that the duration of menopause varies from five to ten years and sometimes longer. I know that my menopause has a few years to go because I am now starting to experience new symptoms. My skin is drying, age spots are appearing, my eyes feel scratchy, my hair is drying and there is an unusual amount of hair left in my hair brush these days. I wasn't blessed with a smooth, soft skin and I was quite lined by my mid thirties so these extra lines are not so worrying for me. I didn't realise that drying would also occur internally. Dr Bev has said that oestrogen pessaries are effective because they provide oestrogen to the vagina and I will try these when I feel I need them.

Of all my menopause symptoms, anxiety has been the worst. I don't believe mine is as bad as some people experience and I have not had depression or panic attacks. It is mild, but it sits in my stomach most times. Simon suggested it was insecurity over him, completely unjustified, he added. But it is not that. I have been through one relationship break-up and went through all the insecurity then. Two ghastly years of my life falling apart; I made sure that I never felt insecure again. I know Simon loves me and there is nothing more Simon could do in our relationship to make it better. No, it's not that. I wish I knew the reason. I never felt this way before menopause; the anxiety appeared with my last period. I haven't explored all avenues and Simon thinks I should talk to a naturopath or herbalist. I think he's right.

Karen has now seen a naturopath for her anxiety and she is trying a herbal combination of hypericum (sometimes known as St John's wort), kava kava and valerian. She said that generally, although not every day, she feels calmer and is able to sleep better. 'An extra hour or two strung together makes the world of difference.' There have been other recommendations, but Karen wants to try solutions one at a time, to give her body a chance to tell her if something is working or not.

She still finds it difficult to concentrate and has reduced the size of her business. Simon is her saviour. He said to me on the phone that he can hardly wait for this book to be out so that he can read what other women are doing about their menopause. I told him that I thought he was going through this menopause as much as Karen.

You better believe it, was his reply.

RHONDA'S STORY

Rhonda is now sixty-eight years old. Her menopause was not the usual journey, starting very early and aggravated by long-term medications. But what is usual? Everyone has their particular set of circumstances.

I am so relieved that I am regaining a normal lifestyle that I feared I had lost. I now realise that menopause isn't the bogeyman (or woman) that will go on tormenting me forever. As my doctor said, 'You will come out of it at some stage. We're just not sure exactly when.'

My menopause has been a long and complicated one. I was given a nickname during those turbulent years – 'Menopause Rhonda'. She was someone who created conflict in a car park and in the supermarket; she had uncontrollable rages and would burst into deep sobs. I should explain that I am, by nature, a quiet and shy person and have spent most of my life caring for my large family. Love, security and support are high on my list and I have never been one to create a scene. But at sixty-six years of age – yes, that old – I plunged into menopausal madness. It seemed that overnight my timid personality changed and was replaced (and controlled) by an erratic creature from hell. I shouted and screamed at everyone, I was extremely emotional.

I had been on and off HRT for many years and at sixty-five my partner noticed that I was having difficulty in getting my thoughts down on paper and sometimes I couldn't find the right word when we were talking. I felt as though I had to trawl through my brain to complete my sentence. We were both worried and after seeing the results of an EEG, my doctor advised me that I had had a minor stroke. He also said that I was to stop HRT immediately. It was not advice but an order! I was apprehensive because I had already had several breaks from HRT, mainly due to the media reports about the risks. During these HRT-free times I had temper tantrums and tears. I was a mother of six school-age children but felt like a rebellious teenager again. Hot flushes plagued me continually, and sleepless nights contributed to general confusion. I had the usual responsibilities of a mother: cooking, cleaning and washing while the children were at school, then helping with homework, answering their questions, listening to their problems, all of them jostling for my attention. I could not afford to be off HRT and yet this was what the doctor was ordering. And instead of six children, I now had twelve grandchildren! In place of HRT I took Promensil, a mild natural alternative which I hoped would work. It didn't.

Before I go any further with my story, I am going to take you back. A long way back. When I married Bob we lived with my parents. Bob and I were in love and wanted to raise a family. While living with my parents our first children were born – twin girls. I had a lot to learn but after three months I was getting into the swing of things. Then I fell pregnant again. 'Bob's a sex maniac,' my mother said to her friend. 'He's got Rhonda expecting again.' We are a Catholic family and relied upon the rhythm method to plan our family. With three babies in my arms, Bob and I tried to be more careful. However, our second son was born two years later and I thought I was so clever producing two girls and two boys!

We were still living with my parents but soon found a big old house to rent on massive grounds. The children thought we lived in a park! And I loved being mistress of my own house. It was when our fifth child was born that I started to feel the stresses of looking after a large family. It was difficult to go for a walk, and shopping was a nightmare. In his work as a policeman Bob worked shifts and this, too, was difficult for both of us. Can you imagine trying to keep five children quiet in the middle of the day while their dad tried to sleep? Sometimes I was left alone at night while Bob was on duty and I had to handle colicky and restless babies on my own. It was not an easy time and I was missing the help from my parents who had always been there for me and the children when we all lived together. So I was feeling quite worn out when my father died suddenly from a heart attack at the age of fifty-nine. Dad had been my rock and I was devastated. We were a very close family – you don't live under the same roof with your parents, your husband and children if you are not close!

It was taking me a long time to accept his death, and with my family commitments and Mum now on her own, I felt all the responsibilities and sadness weighing heavily upon me. It was around this time that I made an appointment to see my doctor. When I walked into his office, his face paled. 'Oh, Rhonda, you're not pregnant again?'

'No. Not yet!' I said and managed a weak smile. 'But I'm just not coping very well. I'm miserable and really missing Dad.'

'I know you are,' he said kindly. 'I don't know how you manage. Five small children! And you're only twenty-seven . . .' He shook his head and prescribed antidepressants. I asked no questions and started on this course. They helped to get me through the long days, and I continued taking them for several years, often moving on to stronger ones. This was forty years ago, when patients did not question their doctor's advice.

We had bought our first home and were moving again. We moved in on Mother's Day and the excitement of having our own house lifted my spirits. Mum liked the idea of a close community and she moved to a caravan park close to us. We were all enjoying establishing our new homes and making new friends and it wasn't long before I was pregnant with our sixth child. In addition to being a police officer, Bob now took on two extra jobs to support us.

For the next three years I managed motherhood very well. We were very happy, albeit extremely busy, and I tackled the everyday chores with gusto. Bob and I had always wanted a large family and now we had one. After the birth of my sixth child I decided not to rely upon the rhythm method and started on the pill. I had no trouble but after a short time I began to have heavy break-through bleeding and a lot of pain between periods. I went to my doctor to ask why this was happening.

'Your uterus is hanging on by a thread,' he said after examining me. 'You will need a repair operation or a hysterectomy.' I was quite shocked. I had always prided myself on being a strong and healthy person whose pregnancies and six births had been trouble-free. I sat feeling very apprehensive about a 'repair' job. What did that mean?

'Rhonda, I would recommend a hysterectomy in your case,' continued my doctor. 'You are very fertile and likely to have a baby every year,' and he shuddered at the thought. I went home and Bob and I talked it over. We felt blessed to have our six children, but they were enough to manage, both physically and financially. It wasn't difficult to decide a hysterectomy would be best. A 'repair' job was more complicated and risked the chance of a relapse and needing to be done again. A hysterectomy was more straightforward and it eliminated the chance of another pregnancy.

I had the hysterectomy and six weeks later my menopause started. I was thirty-five. I want you to remember that I was still blindly taking antidepressants. I just kept getting the prescription filled and no doctor checked whether I still needed them. They were dished out like lollies.

For the first few weeks after my hysterectomy I rested and followed my doctor's instructions. Bob did all he could, despite being on shift work in the police force and doing his extra two part-time jobs. We had generous neighbours who helped by cooking meals, doing my washing and ironing, and running in to check I was okay. We were all in the same boat, living in a new suburb, struggling with young families and everyone helped each other when illness struck or another need presented itself. I recovered well but after six weeks started to experience hot flushes. I had no idea what was happening at first and the sweats increased in intensity and frequency. I hated people looking at me and asking what was wrong. I was shy and embarrassed and couldn't explain.

Off I went to my doctor again. He knew exactly what was happening and told me that I had started early menopause and wrote out a prescription for HRT. He said that I would most likely need to take HRT from now on. For years I continued with antidepressants and HRT, both being given to me without any checkup or review. I took myself off HRT a couple of times when I read in the paper about the risks but during these times menopause affected my emotions severely, and I returned.

In my early forties I had six teenagers. The boys were easygoing, but the girls! Pre-menstrual tension, broken hearts, moods and a continual need for comfort all took its toll. Bob had to retire from the police force due to a back problem that needed surgery and while he was recuperating I went to work. I felt the strain both physically and mentally so my antidepressants were increased and I now added sleeping pills to my bulging medicine cabinet. Arthritis was appearing in my hands and knees and I was diagnosed with an underactive thyroid. More medications!

Life continued to pull me from all sides. One by one the children experienced life away from home, some returning when they realised it wasn't as easy as they thought. Mum, now in her mid eighties, came to live with us, and Bob's health declined. At one stage a daughter returned home to recover from surgery, Mum suffered a stroke and Bob was ill with heart problems. I had thought of putting up a sign on the front door: 'Rhonda's Private Hospital'.

I cared for Mum for seven years before she passed away. Two years later, Bob died from liver cancer. We had been married for forty-two years. The feeling was unreal. Even with a busy life of work, grown-up children and now grandchildren, I felt very empty and lonely.

Let me bring you back to the present when I was ordered to stop HRT after my stroke at sixty-five. The year before my stroke I had decided to take charge of my life and had stopped taking antidepressants. I had been on many different tablets for many years and knew they were having a bad effect on my health. I had for some time felt that I was going through life in a mental fog and so, gradually, and under medical supervision, I weaned myself off these pills. It was not without its side effects but I was coping. The symptoms of insomnia, mood swings, poor memory and general confusion that had been under control for thirty years, all returned when I had to stop HRT. Night became a torture of wakefulness and sweats. I had unbearable skin-crawling itchiness and nothing gave relief. It was all too much for me to bear – and for anyone else. I was referred to the Women's Health Centre and saw a female doctor who specialised in my issues. She understood what I was going through.

'Stopping long-term antidepressants and HRT is putting an enormous stress on you,' she said. Then with a wry smile she said, 'What sane person would come off antidepressants and then cut their legs from under them by coming off long-term HRT in the middle of summer? It's like jumping out of a lifeboat in the middle of an ocean without knowing how to swim!'

Because Promensil did not alleviate the menopause symptoms for me, she advised trying Remefemin. I started on the maximum dose but I'm now down to the minimum and it has been effective although I occasionally get a hot flush. She said that the antidepressants I had been on were old-fashioned and doing me more harm than good. However, she felt I still needed help with my emotions and advised a mild antidepressant, Avanza, and it has provided a gradual improvement.

'You must regain some sort of decent sleep routine, Rhonda. You should rest more through the day if possible. Maybe try and cut down your commitments. Sleep is very important to our general health not only in a physical sense by giving us more energy, but also mentally and emotion- ally. If you are still awake at midnight then you can take a Stilnox sleeping tablet,' she said. I began to get some nights of pretty good sleep and now I only occasionally need the tablet.

'It's important to look at menopause in a positive light, Rhonda,' she often reminded me. 'It can be the beginning of a new and valuable stage of life. It's a time to stop and look at our lifestyle. Care for ourselves a bit better, put ourselves first sometimes and not the family as most of us do.' I saw her every three weeks for a checkup and really enjoyed these discussions.

I took her advice and she was right. I hired a treadmill, joined Weight Watchers and made some definite improve- ments in my fitness. I bought a couple of meditation and relaxation CDs and forced myself to sit in a comfy chair, with eyes closed, phone off the hook, and listen to the soft music and words of wisdom. The result of just ten minutes of this 'time out' is felt for a long period and I value this wonderful release. All these things help to give me a positive outlook and make it easier to cope with any minor menopause symptoms. The mood swings have gone and I am a much nicer person than at this time last year. In fact, I am so much better that the very bad times are a distant memory. Thankfully, 'Menopause Rhonda' has left the building!

I cannot end my story without telling you that I share my life with a kind, gentle and affectionate man, Geoff. We met about four years ago when I was sixty-four. He has been by my side through my stroke, lived with 'Menopause Rhonda', encouraged and praised every little improvement and he gives me so much support, love and respect. I have six children, twelve grandchildren and Geoff. I am very lucky.

Since Rhonda has been going to the Women's Health Centre where she had her medical history and medications assessed, and now continually monitored, she is on the road to a better quality life. Rhonda's children are all adults with their own children and gatherings are a huge event. She is the matriarch of her family.

JULIA'S STORY

Julia was a school teacher with two school-aged children when her menopause started. She also supported her husband in his busy career, attending many social functions as well as entertaining clients in their home. Julia's menopause had just started when her husband suddenly left her, with little explanation. Her symptoms increased and her health faltered.

The audience dissolves into waves of laughter. Menopause the Musical is a hit with my middle-aged Brisbane sisterhood. I sit feeling hot under the collar, fidgeting in my seat, uncomfortable with the realities of sagging flesh and the incontinence pads being flung out at the audience. Instead of enjoying this funny show, it brings all the memories back . . .

'Your blood pressure is up today, Julia,' Dr Tony said, looking at me over steel-framed half glasses. 'Anything wrong?'

'Just some bad news I got this morning, I guess.' I stared at the wall ahead.

'Want to talk about it? Anything I can do?' He gently placed a hand on my shoulder.

'No, well yes,' I reconsidered. 'There is something. Can you give me some tranquillisers. I think I need them,' I blurted out and tears filled my eyes. Tony wrote out a prescription asking me to call him if there were any side effects. His voice was soothing and there was concern in his tone. I was to phone him at the end of the week to get the results of my Pap smear. Fifteen minutes later I'd bought the tablets, swallowed a white pill and tried to convince myself I was fine. I walked down the street, looking at every woman of my age. Do you have hot flushes? Do you suffer from anxiety attacks? Are you menopausal? Has your husband asked for a separation? I wanted to scream at them. Only that morning, Paul had stood looking out the window to where his new, black MGB stood, a little two-seater, that loudly declaimed his mid-life crisis. He had just announced he wanted to leave me.

'Why?' I stammered. My heart raced, or had it stopped? 'We've been good together; we have two beautiful children,' I reasoned. His answer was cruel.

'I don't like the way you dress, the way you do your hair. I don't like the way you look any more,' he said, eyeing me up and down. He picked up the shiny new keys and headed for the door. A hot flush washed over me, sweat clinging to my dress. Oh no, not now. Panic rose in my belly and I struggled to get the next words right.

'I didn't marry you, Paul, for your looks, your hairstyle or your clothes. I loved you, do love you.' But the door closed behind him. I rushed to a mirror to see what Paul could no longer stand. I saw a slim, attractive woman in her late forties, maybe not dressed in the height of fashion, but well-groomed. I also saw a supportive wife, standing by her husband and his career, keeping an immaculate home, paying the bills, saving for holidays, bringing up two children. I had always been there for him. And now, just when life was becoming tricky for me and I needed him, he wanted out.

There was no reconciliation. Married life had become boring and predictable for Paul. He sat in his MGB like a squashed sardine, worried that his thinning hair might blow off. And a new woman sat in the passenger seat. Emma and Sam were at school, and as shocked as I was when their father left. They, too, were confused, angry and needing support. I was forty-seven years old and had just commenced menopause. Initially I was in denial of the symptoms. I quietly removed the bed covers when I was burning up; I'd even given up drinking a single glass of wine with dinner as I could feel how flushed my face became after just a few sips. Now alone, hot flushes, night sweats, accompanying insomnia and fears became my world. I worked within the Education Department, dealing with people all day. Exhaustion affected my concentration, tears reduced me to a child and I became claustrophobic. I didn't want to socialise as I struggled through the maze of menopausal changes, but life had to go on.

I took refuge in Prozac, an antidepressant. It was necessary to take it early in the morning or I would be up all night and hyperactive. On reflection, hormone replacement therapy might have been more effective. As it was, sleep was elusive. I know menopause is connected to insomnia, not only due to hot flushes, but I was also plagued by dreams. Pathetic dreams that I wish I could have controlled. Predictable ones of not being able to find my wedding ring or looking in the wardrobe and finding it empty. Panic attacks in my sleep.

I talked about it to Tania, my cousin from Sydney. We were born four days apart and have had very similar lives with wayward husbands. Tania was also suffering panic attacks, but these occurred usually when she was on the long train journey to work. This was irrational, but we both agreed, more controllable than my dreams. Tania urged me to see my doctor about HRT. It had controlled her panic attacks but she had had side effects. Every time she began a course of tablets, she developed lumps in her breasts. Although they were benign, understandably they bothered her. That was enough to turn me off.

During this period I lost weight. Not only was I struggling to keep myself together, I was extra busy caring for my children. I felt guilty that their father regarded me as inadequate, that I'd let them down by not being good enough in his eyes. I didn't think about food for me, my appetite was poor and I could barely swallow. It was only when my best friend, Robyn, forced me onto the bathroom scales that I read 48.5 kilograms. Ten kilos had vanished! I was astonished that I hadn't even noticed. I was like an automaton, just moving forward, mechanically, trying to keep everything as normal as possible for Emma and Sam. Part of my problem was keeping up the pretence that everything was fine. My marriage had ended, but I was fine. I was menopausal, but I was fine. Only in the evenings, when all was quiet and I was alone, did I give in to how my body was feeling: anxious, lethargic, and hot and sweaty even in winter.

Robyn was concerned and said that I was getting 'cabin fever'. It was an effort for me to get up in the morning let alone face a social engagement, and I refused any of her suggestions. But she persisted and eventually I was dragged off to single's events. At one such occasion I was introduced to a charming Englishman and we soon recognised our kindred souls and retreated for our own version of *Saturday*

Night Fever. A stable relationship developed with Charles and my life, at long last, started to settle down. I could be completely honest with him. No covering up, no hiding, no pretending. He listened to my story and lived with my menopause. He even sought information on the internet and in books so he could help.

Then, when I turned fifty-three, I bled continuously for several weeks. I made an appointment to see my doctor.

'I think it's just my system working it out,' I suggested. 'Hopefully the end of my menopause.' When the results of tests were known my doctor said, 'It's a bit more serious than you thought, Julia. You've got endometrial cancer. You were right to come and see me when you did; it's early detection, but it'll require a hysterectomy.'

The operation was successful, my health improved, and gradually time had done some healing so that I could get on with my life.

. . . Menopause the Musical *is drawing to a close. I tune into the final song, its theme predictably about how change can be good. What an over-simplification! If only life was a musical, I think to myself wryly.*

Julia's menopause clashed with her marriage breakdown. Just when she needed understanding, support and love to help her through menopause she was rejected. Perhaps as a consequence, her menopause affected her more than it might have done. Coping with endometrial cancer tested all her mental power and physical strength. Although she has tried natural therapies they have not been successful in controlling her hot flushes and insomnia. She takes Livial, a synthetic hormone treatment, which helps. She is concerned about long-term effects and has tried to live without it, but her symptoms return along with the misery.

Julia married Charles and they share a very happy life together. His love and understanding encourages her to move forward and to pursue new interests and ambitions.

I FOUND A POEM

I turned fifty
a day or so ago
and avoided the thought
but in my bath
I found a poem —
it was something about a body
that responded to its days
like a well-oiled machine
with parts rusty
bitten
sharp
edgy
and beneath the unexpected softness
and fall
a power
with no name,
and hands that moved
with precision
and grace
an ecstasy
of exactitude, and
something about a brain
and a heart

that embraced the dragon
and saw how the labouring hours
that created the house made the home,
and eyes that can see in the baby
the man and the woman
and in them
the child.
But I've forgotten
exactly
how it went.

Rhonda Cotsell

ANNETTE'S STORY

Annette is married to John and they have two adult children. In her third year of menopause she was finding full-time work too stressful and took the opportunity of long-service leave after which she returned to a part-time position. Heavy and irregular bleeding prompted her to start investigating the right solutions to her menopausal problems, but she discovered that the medical profession often provided conflicting information.

THAT WORD

It seemed odd at first not to be having periods. But I don't miss them one iota! I don't think about not being 'all there' or 'unwomanly'. In fact it is fantastic not to have to worry about them and when I'm walking down the supermarket aisle I bypass all the feminine hygiene products with a gleeful smile. No more flooding or intermittent bleeding. You bloody bewdy! Of course, getting to that stage is not always easy.

The word 'menopause' means the last menstrual period. If only it was one last period, but alas it signifies a time span that is indeterminable. Millions of women have a more colourful description of that word! I do note, however, that the word starts with 'men'. It doesn't seem fair that men don't suffer this particular 'pause' in their lives.

Although they don't get away with it completely; they do have to put up with symptoms and all the vagaries of this phase in a woman's life. For better or worse could have been coined for these times in our lives.

For eight or nine years I had been suffering from heavy bleeding and had seen three gynaecologists. I was given some tablets to help slow the flow and took them for three months. They didn't help. Not only did I continue to bleed three weeks after a period, I also felt bloated and had an outbreak of pimples. I returned to the gynaecologist and we discussed an endometrial ablation, a scraping of my Fallopian tubes, which I considered but decided against. He suggested a hysterectomy, cutting me across the abdomen because I had a large uterus. But I wasn't ready for that either. I was still getting regular monthly periods but they were lasting six to seven days and then some months I would get some slight bleeding a week later. In some months I was bleeding for up to three weeks.

When I was forty-eight I decided to see another gynae-cologist. A blood test showed that I was perimenopausal – that in-between state on the journey to menopause, ending with the final destination of post-pausal. The test showed my levels of hormones were slightly down and that I was anaemic. A course of iron tablets restored my iron level. Besides the blood test, I was experiencing my first menopausal symptoms. I was having the occasional hot flush. They never really bothered me. I would suddenly feel warm, fan my face and they were gone in about ten minutes. I had a sore hip and knew that joint and muscle pain could be a menopause symptom. My breasts were unusually sore. Normally I would get tenderness five to seven days before my period which disappeared when my period started. But this changed to breast soreness two weeks before a period and sometimes continued after my period had finished. I had to wear a stretchy sport bra during the day and to bed. I had to be careful not to knock or bump my breasts and my husband was banned from touching them. One time I thought I had mastitis and used a hot wheat bag which provided relief.

My anxiety increased. I have been fortunate to have had good health but when I was faced with routine medical tests, x-rays, ultrasounds and so forth, I became anxious, wondering what the results would be, thinking of all the negative possibilities. I also noticed that I was having palpitations. This would occur when I was resting, sitting on the bus or watching TV. And this, in turn, increased my anxiety.

I had stress incontinence, my libido dropped and later I had vaginal dryness. This last symptom I found the most upsetting. I felt as if my youth was being sucked out of me and I was becoming old and dried up. I would sometimes lie in bed with my husband asleep next to me and silently cry. I looked the same, but I knew my body was starting to deteriorate. This was the beginning of my slow decline into the blue-rinse brigade and I was having trouble adjusting. It doesn't seem right that while the vagina dries up, there's an increase in incontinence. Not a fair trade off!

I started to research the Net to find as much information as I could on menopause. At this stage my symptoms were not too debilitating and I wanted to be informed and prepared. I started a list of the various foods and their vitamin/mineral contents and which ones are needed for all-round health. I learnt that phytoestrogens are naturally occurring compounds found in plants that are similar to the female hormone oestrogen. I also discovered information about the Mirena, an IUD which releases hormones and is recommended for some women with heavy periods. I had two friends who successfully used this method and who now do not have any monthly periods. This sounded like a good solution for me.

TO WOMB OR NOT TO WOMB, THAT IS THE QUESTION

I made an appointment to see a female gynaecologist. My husband came with me as he is good at thinking of questions to ask and would be aware of the options so we could discuss them rationally together. It's useful to have another person with you to remember all the details as it's easy to forget what you have been told. After examining me and discussing my particular circumstances, she recommended a hysterectomy as the best option.

'I would perform a laparoscopy, making three small incisions here,' she explained. 'Your womb is large, Annette, and your incontinence is caused by the weight of these fibroids pressing on your bladder. Removing your womb should take the weight off your bladder. There's a bit of thickening in your womb and if you decide not to proceed with a hysterectomy I would want to do a biopsy as soon as possible.' She explained the procedure thoroughly and I felt confident in her ability. I also had my fingers crossed! I made my decision and was booked to have the operation.

BRING ON THURSDAY

It was with great pleasure and a touch of serendipity that I noted in my diary the date of the first day of my last menstruation – 4 March 2006. Full stop, period! In six days

I would have my laparoscopic hysterectomy. Never again would I have to take large packets of pads on holiday or stuff them into my bra and sneak off to the toilet at work or excuse myself from meetings in order to change. No more panty liners in case I coughed or started to bleed unexpectedly. No longer would I be a prisoner of my womb, my hormones or my bladder.

No more Lady Macbeth for me!

For all my positive thinking and determination, I felt challenged by insidious anxiety. But I kept focused on the wonderful benefits and freedom and pressed the 'delete' button on anxiety. I kept visualising myself on holiday, going out without ever having to consider my body's needs. I saw myself jumping up with my fist in the air shouting, 'Yahoo. Yes, yes, I did it!'

THE DAWNING OF THE DAY

I drove myself to hospital, calm and relaxed. The mind is a powerful tool! I was checked by the anaesthetist and given theatre stockings which reminded me of the ones I used to wear in the seventies with hot pants. I had to wait for several hours before the operation and I started to get a bit antsy. What was it I said about the mind? The last thing I remembered was a metallic taste in my mouth and looking up at the theatre lights. I awoke around seven in the evening. I was wheeled to a private room and my husband walked in.

'How do you feel, love?' he said taking my hand.

'Not bad. A bit tired. There's not much pain,' I managed to say.

The operation was successfully performed via a vaginal laparoscopy and I only had two small incisions in my lower abdomen and a tiny cut in my bellybutton. It's quite fantastic what medical techniques are available to us today. I had no after-effects from the anaesthetic. The catheter, draining tube and drip were removed later in the morning and after lunch I was able to get up. I only required a Panadol twice a day for the pain, such as it was. The operation was performed on the Thursday night and I was home Saturday afternoon. Over the next couple of days a nurse visited to check on my recovery and later to remove the stitches.

Within two weeks I was able to get around normally. I wandered around my back garden, enjoying the sunshine and felt very proud of myself. Because I had my ovaries removed and therefore would not be producing oestrogen, my gynaecologist prescribed Premarin, oestrogen supplements. She said that the supplement would assist in reducing the menopausal symptoms. I started on two Premarin tablets daily after the operation and they worked well, initially. I wasn't experiencing any menopausal symptoms and my vaginal fluid increased noticeably. The sore area I had had in my hip for over a year also disappeared.

THAT WORD (AGAIN!)

At my six week post-operative checkup with the gynaecologist, I mentioned that I had started to get prickly/itchy feelings in my legs, mainly at night in bed but sometimes during the day. I would also be woken during the night with pins and needles in my hands. She suggested I drop Premarin to one tablet per day. I tried that for a month but didn't feel much different other than my vagina became a little dry again, so I decided to go back to two.

Then I started to experience light-headedness and an unusual feeling in my head, mainly around the base of my skull. It was a burning, prickly feeling. I didn't take much notice of it at first until it occurred more frequently and I was worried that I might pass out. I rang my gynaecologist and asked her if it was a side effect of the Premarin but was informed it wasn't and that I should go to my local GP.

A visit to my GP showed that my blood pressure was up a bit which surprised me. I had never had any problems before and my blood pressure was fine after the operation. I was advised to cut back on caffeine and alcohol to see if that had any effect on the palpitations I was also having. I went home and started to walk more regularly to relax and try to reduce my blood pressure.

On a second visit my blood pressure was up a bit more, as was my cholesterol. This also surprised me as I eat lots of salad, fruit and wholemeal bread. I don't spread margarine on my bread or eat much fried food or cakes. So what was going on?

'I'm not keen on you taking HRT,' the doctor said. 'I think if the menopausal symptoms can be managed in other ways it would be better if you stopped Premarin.'

'But I don't have my ovaries and I'm not producing any oestrogen, which I believe I need,' I said doubtfully, now worried that Premarin might be affecting my blood pressure.

I reduced Premarin back to one tablet again and during the week waves of anxiety washed over me. I would sit down and try to talk rationally to myself, a strategy which had worked in the past when I was feeling anxious. I was getting worried that I would give myself a heart attack or stroke. I started to think that maybe I was bleeding in my head because a feeling of warmth would creep up my body and rise up into my head, causing an odd sensation.

During a shopping outing with my sister, I had an anxiety attack. I could feel myself suddenly starting to get anxious for no reason, with a feeling of wanting to escape. I kept talking and looking at things, hoping it would pass. We had some lunch but I still felt uneasy amongst a lot of people. My sister has also experienced anxiety attacks so she understood what I was feeling. Before lunch finished I was feeling better.

There were other concerns. My appetite dropped and I was having trouble getting to sleep. My thoughts were constantly racing around, jumping from one thing to another and usually negative. I could not relax and as soon as I tried to change the thought to something positive, it vanished in a flash, replaced by another negative one. When I did manage to get to sleep I would suddenly wake in the middle of the night feeling tense with my heart racing. I would get up, have a glass of cold water, stand on a cold floor or sit and do some deep breathing until my heart slowed. When I returned to bed it was often difficult to get back to sleep and I would be awake for a couple of hours.

I made two appointments to discuss the situation with my GP and gynaecologist. Both professionals were giving me different opinions and this was not helping me to make the best decision. My husband and I were also going on a two-week holiday before I returned to work and I wanted to get myself straight before leaving. I didn't want to be away from home feeling anxious and unable to sleep. I even made sure that I knew where a hospital was, close to where we would be staying, just in case!

My blood pressure had risen even further and my heart rate was very high when I visited my GP. He started me on Avapro for my blood pressure and I asked for something to help me get my sleeping pattern back to some normality.

My gynaecologist listened to my story when I next saw her and she felt confident that it was due to a low level of oestrogen. 'There's a lot of misinformation about hormone replacement therapy and many GPs don't understand HRT,' she said. 'Let's go through the signs and symptoms of oestrogen deficiency.' These included feeling light-headed, insomnia, anxiety, depression, crawling feelings under the skin, all of which I had been experiencing. I could see the pattern.

'I'll write a letter to your GP, Annette, explaining things to him and why I think you should stay on HRT. Because you're only fifty-one I truly believe that you should be taking oestrogen. It's less than what is in the pill and the benefits are that it protects your heart from cardiovascular disease and it maintains good bone density,' she said. 'As you're finding it difficult to manage on the tablets, I would recommend you try the patches. I'm sure you'll feel a lot better within twenty-four hours.' I left the consultation feeling more confident.

My husband and I drove straight to the chemist to fill the prescription and when I got home I slapped the patch on my backside as quickly as possible. The following morning we packed our car and I felt a psychological boost, now that I was armed with my new medications. However, it took longer than I expected before I started to feel any better. I was trying hard not to spoil the holiday but I felt tense in my back and anxiety still crossed my path. After settling in to a cabin I said, 'Let's go for a walk and check out the place.' We found a track that meandered along the foreshore, past a marina and culminated with a climb through native vegetation to a panoramic lookout.

Normally I would have enjoyed this experience, but I had to constantly force myself to focus on the surroundings to ease my anxiety. I couldn't understand why I wasn't relaxed or why my thoughts were out of control.

I hadn't told John about my anxiety attacks but I had mentioned that I was getting waves of anxiety. 'Just try to relax,' he advised and held my hand. He tried to keep me chatting, which helped somewhat, but my comments were generally short. I am not a person who discusses my problems or fears easily. I was somewhat concerned I was losing the plot and John must have been thinking the same. I didn't want to be constantly complaining. People who whine are not pleasant company. When we did talk it was only temporary relief. I was reluctant to eat out and was uneasy about being away from the cabin for long periods of time. I preferred to make meals or buy something and bring it back. I guess I wanted to be near help if I needed it. I had a fear of heights and walking over a low bridge made me feel uncomfortable. Climbing open stairs was a challenge. After stopping at sight-seeing places I was impatient to leave. On the way back John suggested we wander around the marina.

'I don't want to,' I replied.

'We can get a coffee and enjoy the view,' he said.

'I want to go back to the cabin. I don't feel like walking anymore,' I responded.

He could see I was hesitant and said sharply, 'I've never known you to have such a negative attitude. Just relax will you!'

'I can't help it. If I could relax I would. I don't like being like this,' I answered angrily. We were both perplexed by my behaviour.

It took about three days before I started to feel better and by the fifth day I was eating more and starting to relax, although I was not sleeping well. In the end we had a good holiday but I think it would have been disastrous without my medication.

LIGHT AT THE END OF THE TUNNEL

It has taken nearly five months to get my oestrogen dose right. I am now on Estraderm patches and they are changed twice a week. I don't have the prickly/itchy feelings in my legs as I had with Premarin. The patches are great because I don't have to remember to take a tablet every day. I am still on tablets to keep my blood pressure right and my cholesterol is back to normal. My breasts are no longer sore – a major relief – and the heart palpitations have settled down. I am able to drink a little coffee now and have a glass of wine without causing any problems. My bladder control has improved. I went to a show recently and sat through the performance for an hour without having to slip away to the toilet. Before the operation I would not have lasted. My mojo has made a slight reappearance for its last encore and there is also an increase in the vaginal fluid – no more thoughts of 'old hag' in the making. She can wait in the wings until this current show winds up!

Annette advises women to be proactive about their menopause. She is on HRT and plans to gradually decrease the dose over time. Her gynaecologist has said that she could continue for another ten years which she said would protect Annette from osteoporosis. Annette has noticed that she is less willing to make decisions and gets anxious if she is not organised, but finds that yoga helps her to keep a positive mind and aids relaxation.

Over the last few years Annette and John have developed a taste for Moroccan and Indian food. Both these cultures use lentils, chick peas and legumes which provide phytoestrogens. She continues to eat plenty of fruit, vegetables and sprouting seeds and grains.

PAT'S STORY

Pat is a professional playwright, puppeteer and community artist. She is married to Paul, a draftsman, and their work has taken them to all corners of Australia. Pat's menopause started in her late forties, just prior to packing up their travelling motorhome to move halfway across Australia. She tells her story by referring to her diary notes written during those years. She is a meticulous woman and found her symptoms debilitating.

23 January 1994: I couldn't concentrate today. At 10 am I gave up trying to achieve anything, so I left my desk and went for a long walk, hoping to oxygenate the brain. Working from home has its advantages!

15 February: The principal rang from one of the up-market private schools wanting to book my show. He said that the drama teacher wants to introduce the students to puppetry. We set a date and some times. I couldn't find my diary until after we had hung up and by then I'd forgotten the dates and times. I rang him back with an invented lame reason to get the dates again.

18 February: Still can't concentrate and I seem to be feeling menstrual but I can't be according to the calendar. In fact

I'm feeling premenstrual all the time and it's scary. I don't know what it means. I've never really minded feeling premenstrual because it only lasts a few days. And the trick to surviving it has always been to try and not achieve too much. And to try and not bite everyone's heads off. But now that I feel like this all the time I don't know how to handle it. Am I always going to be like this?

23 February: Mum rang and said she's been given an appointment to see the surgeon. She asked if I would go with her because she's afraid she might forget what the surgeon says. I couldn't tell her why I thought this was funny. Decided to buy a notebook to write down what the surgeon says.

26 February: I'm mortified! Horribly mortified! Went to Julia's house (the play's director). Arrived promptly as expected at 2 pm. She wanted to discuss the play's progress and a few other things. Her brother answered the door and said she was out and that she'd been expecting me on the previous Tuesday. I must have written down the wrong date. What must she think of me? She seems to be a stickler for punctuality and details and I'm usually so professional about those things.

5 March: After giving three shows a day for three days in a big school I'm completely bushed. I couldn't even unload the puppets from the car when I got home. Instead I prostrated myself full length on the couch. Then I noticed that the dishes from last night's meal were still piled on the sink in a congealing tower. At 6 pm Paul and the boys started nosing around in the kitchen wondering what was for tea. I exploded.

'I'm not cooking tonight. Anyone who wants to eat will have to make their own arrangements,' I said gesticulating at the mess in the sink. One part of me likes having the boys home again. Deep down I'm just a sooky mother who likes having her children around. When they first left home it was terrible. I couldn't believe my reaction. I was miserable and depressed. I thought that only happened to people who had nothing else in their lives. Then one by one they came back home again, just as I'd got used to a quiet house and an easier life. Aaargh!

My outburst about cooking set off a squabble between the boys and ended with number two son stomping off and slamming the door. I feel angry with him for acting so childishly but my heart aches for them when the postman brings 'thanks, but no thanks' letters for their job applications. It's so hard for young people to get onto the first rung of the career ladder in 1994. The recession *we had to have* has a lot to answer for.

7 March: Took Mum to see the surgeon. He's a terrible communicator and talked to me over Mum's head as if she's blind and deaf. Evidently the stents that were inserted years ago are no longer viable and will have to be replaced. Mum accepted this news as if it had been handed down by God from the mountain. I was having a particularly bad day and could hardly concentrate on what he was saying. I scribbled everything he said in the notebook. I'm concerned about her having major surgery at eighty and in a frail state of health, and said to her that I think we should discuss it further with the surgeon. She was adamant that if the surgeon thinks she should have the operation then that is what she will do.

8 March: Paul came home from work ashen-faced with news that his drafting contract is coming to an end prematurely. The recession is hitting South Australia and every night on the news we see that yet another factory is closing. I notice that the strain is showing on people's faces in the street. Luckily I've got plenty of work to keep us going for the time being. Paul said that his enforced leisure would give him the opportunity to work on converting the passenger bus that we bought last year to a motorhome.

10 March: My period hasn't come. At forty-eight I can't be pregnant! I mustn't be. The implications don't bear thinking about. I'm virtually the bread winner. And Mum needs me. I dragged myself off to the doctor with a sample of the appropriate bodily fluid.

11 March: I told Paul why I went to the doctor yesterday. He was astounded. His face registered a kaleidoscope of emotions. I told him that in spite of everything I couldn't possibly have a termination. I stated again, 'I just couldn't!' He said he would stand by what ever decision I made and disappeared into the shed to do what men do in these circumstances. Against all logic I start to feel twinges of excitement about the prospect of new life. How mad is that? Me – ultra-practical Pat!

13 March: Back to the doctor to get the results. 'Negative' she told me waiting for my response. 'That's good,' I said, and then I was overwhelmed by a sudden rush of intense disappointment and burst into tears. I felt ridiculous. She said I was probably perimenopausal and took blood for an FSH test to measure the amount of follicle-stimulating hormone in the blood. She explained FSH helps to control

the menstrual cycle and it can help determine whether a woman is menopausal. Then I told her that I couldn't remember anything. 'I can't even follow the plot of *The Bill* on television and I'm moody and short-tempered. It's just not like me,' I said. She looked kind of knowing and gave me several pamphlets on menopause. The symptoms they describe are pretty general, and I suppose I have quite a few of them. She suggested I think about the idea of HRT. 'Definitely not,' I said haughtily. 'That's for people who can't cope with the idea of aging. It's a natural event for goodness sake,' I added sticking to my little prejudices. On the way home I called into the library to get books which will explain more about menopause than the pamphlets have done. One of the books is particularly interesting. Each chapter is written by someone from a completely different culture and talks about the attitude of people towards menopause in that culture. There is a contribution from a Chinese doctor, a Japanese grandmother, an orthodox Western doctor, an alternative Western doctor – and that's all I've read so far. The attitudes are fascinatingly different. One writer talks about the ancient view of the post-menopausal woman who was revered as the Crone or the Wise Woman to whom people turned for advice. Hmmn. Wise woman, eh? An interesting idea. Perhaps I could aspire to that ... enjoy it even. Not that I feel wise today. I just feel confused, tired and strung-out.

16 March: Back to the doctor again for the FSH test results. She said that I am definitely menopausal and probably won't have any more periods. She was wrong about that – my periods started today during a performance.

I got up earlier than usual and drove to a school on the

edge of town. I felt rotten – a shocking cold and hardly any voice. I wasn't sure how I was going to get through the shows. The weather was freezing and the rain was so heavy I had to pull over by the side of the road for a while. Then during the first performance I could tell that my period was starting. Luckily no one noticed. Thank goodness for the puppeteer's black costume!

17 March: Maggie rang and said that although we are both busy we still should make time for our friendship. I agreed and we met for coffee. She looked haggard. 'I'm not sleeping,' she said. 'Bloody night sweats! And then in the day constant hot flushes. Yesterday I had a big one – whoosh – in front of a client. It was so embarrassing. I told the client I was having a power surge!' We laughed until the café staff glared at us. Just before we left the café, I got up to go to the toilet. Didn't quite make it. Now I'm wetting my pants! How degrading. Upset, I told Maggie but she just laughed. I joined in and we left the café doubled over, helpless. I haven't felt so good for months.

18 March: I got home at 4.30 pm after doing two shows at an inner-city school. Paul was dancing around the place, ecstatic. He'd had an offer of work from someone in central Queensland who wanted him to start the job in four months. Paul thinks we should accept the offer and says he could work flat out on the bus conversion and bring our post-retirement travelling plans forward and turn them into a working holiday. He's incredibly excited. I'm too tired to think. Lately I'm having trouble marshalling enough facts in my head to be able to make decisions. I went to bed in a state of mild shock. What Paul proposes is probably a good idea. I can't really tell.

23 June: We decided that Paul should accept the offer so we're leaving for Queensland in a couple of days. After that, who knows?

There's been so much happening in the last few months that I've been too preoccupied to write my diary. Mum's operation was a success, thank goodness, but there was a long period of recovery. She's become very dependent on me and won't have any community volunteers. She thinks a daughter's role in life is to look after her mother and she seems to resent my work. Then Dad had two spells in hospital and the house was like a rehabilitation centre for a while with nurses coming in to shower them, a cleaner and Meals on Wheels. They are back on their feet again, though frail. Their situation has made my decision to go to Queensland agonising but I've left responsibility for them in the hands of my brothers who are perfectly capable of handling the situation. My boys have found flats and although they are delighted for us I think they are the ones now feeling the 'empty nest syndrome'.

The last two days have been filled with frantic activity as we packed up our possessions and put them into storage. Although I'm excited about our big adventure my ability to concentrate is so bad that I've found packing to be an almost insurmountable task. I've been dithering around indecisively and feeling so ashamed of my incompetence that I've developed clever strategies to hide it from the family. I have also been cunning at work: when I've been to meetings I've not always been able to follow what was going on, so I would not ask any questions in case the issue had already been discussed and this had gone over my head. I was *acting* so that I would not look unspeakably foolish.

26 June: Today is the start of our Great Adventure. We're nomads, gypsies, people of the road. As we leave Adelaide, the weather is grey, drizzly and miserable, but we are heading towards sunshine and optimism. Our hearts are high. The problems of the last two years slide away behind us with every passing kilometre.

3 July: We are on the central Queensland coast and have settled into a caravan park. Our motorhome is parked a few metres from the sea. My senses are overwhelmed by the warm air, the stupendous foliage, the sea opal-green and blue, the frangipani hanging on the breeze, the exuberant bougainvillea. Lotus land. The clichés are all true.

10 July: Paul has started work but I've decided to take six months off to rest and acquire a sense of skills for the tropics. Like learning to get in and out of a hammock with dignity.

12 August: A month of rest hasn't had much effect. This morning we drove into town to do the shopping. The scenery and weather were glorious, everything in technicolour, when I burst out, 'It's a terrible day and everything is awful.' Paul looked baffled and asked if I wanted to go back home.

'No! What good would that do?' I snapped. Ten minutes later we were walking around the supermarket and Paul asked how I was.

'Fine. Why?'

16 August: I am really excited today. There's an opportunity for me to instigate a radio project, interviewing twelve local people about their life stories. I've said that I'll do it.

24 August: Went out today to interview a South Sea Islander man about his experiences working in the sugar industry. I found driving to his home on an unfamiliar road incredibly difficult because I felt very light-headed and I had problems concentrating on the traffic, even though there were very few cars on the road! I fumbled with the tape recorder that the radio station lent me. I'm sure the man didn't notice my confusion and his story was fantastic.

27 September: Have finished three more interviews and, although the work is fascinating, I'm barely able to phrase my questions. I bluff my way through and I'm sure no one realises that I'm only just coping by the skin of my teeth. I struggle through the days, hours, even minutes, and in desperation I have made an appointment to see a local GP about HRT.

2 October: I saw a local woman doctor. In the past I've never minded whether my doctor was male or female. The quality I look for is empathy and that we somehow be on the same wavelength. However, as menopause is such an intensely female experience I thought a female doctor would be better. She is young, pretty and bright, newly married. When I sat and tried to tell her my story, groping for words and hardly able to remember the symptoms, I thought she looked at me with a slightly scornful expression. I'm sure she thought I was barmy. We briefly discussed HRT. She said that a patch is now available for both oestrogen and progesterone which I was very pleased to learn. But we didn't talk about the pros and cons of HRT so I'm still very undecided. She has lent me a video and some books. Hopefully they will enlighten me so that I can make a sensible decision.

8 October: Went back to the doctor today and screamed, 'Give me the patch. Now!' I was completely overwhelmed with all the symptoms. So at forty-nine years of age I start on HRT. It's taken a big shift in attitude towards HRT to come to this decision.

17 October: I'm sure that it's not my imagination or the placebo effect but I feel a slight improvement. By no means completely okay – no more than a general lift of wellness.

19 December: I've been on HRT for about two months now and I'm feeling quite a lot better. There's been a dramatic improvement in the bedroom department – not that I thought there was anything amiss before, but I'm wondering if there is a dosage of testosterone in the patch as well! Paul must think he's in heaven!

14 January 1995: Wonderful conclusion to the radio project today. Earlier in the day, I prepared the hall with cups and saucers for the afternoon tea at the conclusion of the presentations and speeches. Such a simple task, but I struggled with organising this. Where to put the china? Here, or over there? I wandered from one end of the room to the other, picking up a cup and not knowing what to do with it. Paul, by now well aware of my limitations, could see that I was becoming unreasonably stressed and offered to help me.

The mayor presented copies of the taped interviews to each participant and to the town's head librarian for the oral history section. The ABC manager said how pleased he was about the project and the mayor said all the right things. Although my concentration still wavers and is a long way from where I would like it to be, when it was time for my speech I stood up and without referring to notes said everything I wanted to say strongly, confidently and with a certain aplomb. I was amazed that I did so well. I suppose there's no business like show business for teaching one to carry things off!

15 February: I needed a new prescription for the patch today so I made an appointment. On my arrival at the doctors' rooms I was informed that I would be seeing a locum doctor. The young, clever, pretty doctor was taking some maternity leave because she was finding her pregnancy challenging. I sat in the waiting room and wondered how *she* was coping and felt an unseemly sense of satisfaction.

The locum asked me how I was managing with the patch saying some people find it unsuitable in the tropics because of perspiration. I said that I would like to continue with it as I thought that the patch was kinder on the liver and I could manage with the humidity.

21 March: Paul's contract finished today. He flew south, 400 kilometres, for a job interview and came back excited with the job in his pocket.

23 May: We are living on yet another idyllic tropical beach in Queensland. We've met some interesting people who have made us feel at home already. My daily routine is pretty limited. I spend the afternoons resting and reading.

30 July: It's been a couple of years since I've had a mammogram so I'm having one today. I had a needle biopsy on a breast lump three years ago, the doctor was being very cautious and there was nothing untoward detected. I'm lumpy again in both breasts but I think this is just hormonal changes.

2 August: Received a letter from BreastScreen, asking me to return for further checking.

7 August: Feeling very anxious and had to have another mammogram. Thankfully, given the all-clear. I took the opportunity to talk to the attending doctor about HRT and said to him that although I felt it was helping my symptoms, it was nevertheless a mixed blessing. He nodded and didn't say much but his expression told me that he very much agreed with this. I left worrying about my breasts and feeling uncertain about HRT.

10 October: It's been a year since I started on HRT. I feel it has enabled me to function better, but I am far from feeling my old self, or rather younger self. I am decidedly uneasy about HRT and know that I should make a decision about whether to continue or not.

3 March 1996: Today I visited the local doctor's surgery. He was away and his locum was a mature woman doctor. That's good, I thought. I said to her that I was thinking of going off HRT and told her about my concerns with breast cancer. I was astonished by her reaction. 'If you do, you may well find yourself in the position of many old ladies who fall and, due to osteoporosis, break their hips. They are a burden to their families and spend many months in hospital at an expense to society.' I was furious. I went home and ripped off the patch.

6 March: An immediate response to my rash action. I'm suddenly deeply depressed and my memory has a five-minute span. My moods swing wildly and, no matter how hard I try not to be, I am horrible to Paul. I'm crying half the day for no reason and I feel the lowest I have felt in my whole life.

8 March: Maggie rang. I was so pleased to hear her cheerful voice. 'How are you and how's your love life?' she quipped, not really expecting an answer to that question. 'Funny you should ask me that today,' I said. 'I've just gone off the patch and all my passion has vanished – completely drained away. I feel lifeless.' Poor Maggie wasn't sure what to say.

I told Paul that my lack of sexual enthusiasm was because of the humidity and heat but I'm sure Paul sensed it is due to menopause. I've tried to explain to him why I'm like I am, but he has already realised, of course, that I'm different and unpredictable. I sense that he has stepped back from the situation because he doesn't fully understand what is going on with me but that he has noted that there are great changes taking place and that his role should be one of support. We had been squabbling a bit because I'm less patient but I can see that he is making a big effort to deal with my moods. Fortunately he's a very adaptable and mature person and that is why he's coping with this difficult situation.

12 March: Before Paul came home from work, I was curled up in the foetal position on the lounge. I felt like an inmate in a nineteenth-century lunatic asylum who has nowhere to go for help. I knew I couldn't go on like this so I visited the local pharmacy to see what alternatives to HRT are available. I started to tell the story to a kind-looking woman behind the counter and became almost incoherent. With great empathy she sat me down on a chair in a quiet spot and brought me a few products. Then she told me about the local naturopath who has a very good reputation and who works hand-in-hand with many of the local doctors.

15 March: I made an appointment with the naturopath. He listened carefully and told me that he has a number of patients in my position and that they find his herbal treatments work well. He prescribed chasteberry and tripholium complex and a progesterone cream. They are hideously expensive and the herbs, which are in liquid form, are vile tasting. The naturopath told me that he thinks I am probably a compulsive achiever! I responded defensively and admitted to being a little driven but think that he is exaggerating.

16 March: I keep thinking about what the naturopath said. Perhaps there's a thin line between having plenty of drive and stepping over the line towards being a compulsive achiever. Although I hate to admit it, I think that he could be right. Perhaps I should think seriously about my approach to things. I know the library has plenty of books in what I scornfully dismiss as the 'self help' section. There may be something appropriate for me. I'll have a browse.

1 May: I'm starting to feel better, although the improvements are not quite as 'wham bam' as conventional HRT. At least when I'm at the shops I can remember what I have gone for. I'm feeling stronger both mentally and physically. And the activity in the bedroom has resumed, albeit at a more sedate pace than the frenzy when I was on the patch.

I found some very good books which have quite a lot of relevance to the way I set goals and have high expectations of myself and so I'm keeping a journal, quite apart from my daily diary, in which I monitor the way I do things. One suggestion is to look at my actions from an outsider's point of view and try and work out plans for modifying my behaviour if I feel this is necessary. Given that I am too flat to work properly at the moment I will see this as an opportunity to 'look within'.

31 July: Paul has another job, in WA. So here we are again on another tropical breeze but in the dry tropics this time with the sky solid cobalt, the water vivid turquoise, the mangroves green and the beach a strip of red sand. The journey from Brisbane to Broome was an amazing adventure.

I decided to visit a local doctor. Although the herbal remedies from the naturopath have been pleasingly effective, I'm experiencing tenderness under one arm and in the side of the breast. The local doctor feels that this is not an acceptable symptom and suggests that I take Remifemin, a natural HRT, which has been used in Germany for thirty years and which works very well for his own wife.

28 October: Remifemin has proved to be very good for me although I have experienced a little tenderness on and off.

May 2007: We are now back home in South Australia where we have built a new house for ourselves in the gorgeous Adelaide Hills and our motorhome has gone to a new pair of adventurers.

I now realise that when Paul and I travelled around Australia, I was on another journey at the same time. This journey took me over rough roads from being a driven, capable, dynamic, goal-orientated person who looked after everyone and everything in my circle, to someone struggling with every aspect in my life. Now, at that journey's destination, I am far less driven and I'm able to *go with the flow*. I'm still dynamic but the dynamism is less in the style of the bull in a china shop. I have a renewed sense of mental vigour and, although I have far less physical energy than I once had, I have the same enthusiasm for life which I felt when I was twelve years old and was looking to life taking me on its exciting course.

Looking back on this journey I can see that I have undergone a complete transformation – physical, emotional, mental and spiritual. Perhaps Nature intends women to take this journey at menopause and, as change can be frightening sometimes, it's no wonder that some of us struggle hard against it. I can see that this journey through menopause has led me to discover a secret land – a place where I now live and which once I knew nothing about. It's the best place I've lived in – ever!

Pat has recently turned sixty. She has a new business guiding others in writing creative life stories. She offers mentoring and editing services and enjoys the challenge of turning history into living words. She still struggles a bit with the notion of people doing things for her, but this is now her new challenge – being able to accept the help.

Pat has had a long menopause journey and some symptoms still linger. Her memory can still be patchy and she relies on her diary and notebook, although they are not useful when she can't find her glasses! She takes no medication for menopause and the tenderness under her arm and around her breast has gone.

Sitting in Pat's home, overlooking deep valleys of stringy-bark gums we ponder the issue of women reaching the rank of 'wise woman'. Pat says, *wisely*, 'I don't know if I have reached that venerable status. That is for others to judge.'

GLENDA'S STORY

Glenda has been married to Kingsley for forty-one years. They have two children and three grandchildren who live in Canada. Glenda is a professional artist and her work can be found around the world with many works commissioned for corporate collections. All proceeds support families, currently nine, through World Vision. Glenda's menopause started at forty-nine when she and her husband were planning a 'sea change'.

My husband had just been offered a 'package' and after twenty years of living in Canada we decided it was time to leave the ice and snow behind us and head back home to Australia. Our children were three and five when we moved there and now they were at university, we hoped they might follow us. They'd both been adamant about retaining their Australian citizenship and so we were quite hopeful. We had aging parents in Australia and we were planning on spending some quality time with them before it was too late.

The house was on the market, the container with our furniture was on the high seas, the dog was in Australia in quarantine and as we drove out of town the first snowflakes of the season were falling. My husband said, 'Time to leave,' and we felt quite smug at the thought of heading first to visit friends in the US, enjoying time in warm Arizona and Houston, then flying from there to England and on to Ireland, while in Canada they were heading into another cold winter.

It had been a hectic few months and trying to pull all the loose ends together hadn't been easy. In addition, for some months I'd been having headaches, stomach cramps, heavy bleeding, sleepless nights, leg cramps and I would often burst into tears for no reason. With the enormous pressure and stress of everything going on in our lives in the months before we left, these symptoms became more severe. I thought it best to visit our friendly GP of twenty years for his help and advice.

Dr Ward said, 'Having known you and your family for the duration of your stay here in Canada, I have to think that you're starting menopause. After all you're almost fifty! Some of your symptoms are quite debilitating and it would certainly be helpful if we could regulate the heavy bleeding and eliminate some of the problems before you head off into the "blue yonder" and find yourself in situations where it's going to be difficult to get medical advice.'

'Rick,' I said, 'my whole life is very uncertain at this point in time; there's so much going on in our lives. I'm feeling hugely emotional about leaving behind my children, friends and my art career … so maybe its just stress causing these problems?'

'Trust me,' he said and gave me one of his famous twinkling smiles, 'all of that might well be true, but your symptoms are definitely menopausal.'

I'd suffered from monthly cramps and heavy bleeding for years, but what I was experiencing now was a real flood. It arrived with a vengeance and could be rather embarrassing. Yet other months it was very light and lasted just a day or so. Before making any decision about HRT solutions, I decided to heed Rick's advice and I attended the clinic's lecture given regularly by their nursing staff.

When I arrived I was quite surprised to find that there were about thirty women gathered, some older, many much younger. There was a variety of literature handed around outlining the symptoms and supposed remedies for menopause, mostly promotional material put out by the pharmaceutical companies. Once the nurse had gone through this with us we were encouraged to ask questions and that's when I realised that many women suffered far worse symptoms than me. While I had occasional hot flushes and night sweats, leg cramps and sleepless nights, often had the sensation of things crawling up my arms, sometimes felt anxious, forgetful, muddle-headed and irritable, some women admitted to having to get up several times a night to shower, change sheets and bed clothes. There were others who admitted to spending their days constantly yelling and screaming at husbands and children, often resorting to violence due to depression, anxiety, irritability and the fact that they couldn't sleep. Some felt they'd become monsters overnight!

There was a lot of discussion about various herbal remedies. Some admitted they'd tried them but hadn't benefited from their use. Others had started taking Premarin and Progesterin; some had side effects, others were thrilled with the results. Some were using vaginal creams, others taking powders, on and on it went. Some had a family history of breast cancer; what should they use? Others had other medical situations affecting their choices. It was all very confusing for me. I found out that oestrogen is the primary hormone responsible for female characteristics. This sounded good, no matronly figure or hairy chin and upper lip for me. A youth pill. Wow! It is also considered important for cardiac and vascular health and helps prevent osteoporosis.

When I went back to visit my doctor I said, 'Rick, I'm totally confused. You know there is a history of heart disease in my family, yet there's been no evidence of breast cancer on my maternal side. If I was your wife, what would you advise?'

'I'd prescribe Premarin and Provera for you without any hesitation. Give it a try and if there are no side effects, then I think it will be helpful for you.'

'Right, let's do it!' I said.

My doctor told me that anything around the uterus – dead cells, mucus, blood – that needs to come away would be shed. This did continue for a few months after I started HRT in pill form and then my periods became very light and eventually just spotty. I had no side effects from the pill although I did gain a little weight, or was that due to all that delicious Cajun food in Houston and the delicious dishes our friends kept pressing on us; or the fact that it was so nice sitting out in the Arizona sunshine sipping a glass of wine in the middle of the day?

We travelled to England, bought a second-hand car at auction and headed over to Ireland. We stayed in some wonderful locations, mainly in the Ring of Kerry renting self-catering accommodation on a weekly basis. We hiked up and over mountains, swam in the lakes, met some wonderful people and in fact loved it so much we agreed to come back the following year and rent a 300-year-old farmhouse for the whole season – from April to the end of September.

During that time I had only experienced very minor menopausal symptoms. Sometimes I'd like to attribute forgetfulness and irritability to menopause, but really I think it's nice to have an excuse sometimes for these short-comings. I sometimes felt hot and flushed, kept having to dangle my feet out of bed in the middle of the night because they felt hot and tingly, and there were the occasional leg cramps, very painful and tender the next day. But generally I felt healthy and content with life.

Back in South Australia we purchased a lovely town-house, within walking distance of the centre of Adelaide, took the dog out of quarantine, the furniture out of storage and set up the property very comfortably. After settling in for a few months and celebrating an early Christmas with our family that year, we gave the dog to friends to care for, rented out the townhouse and returned to Ireland. We'd decided before we got on with the rest of our lives that it would be sensible to get Ireland out of our system. We arrived in Ireland on 1 April, April Fool's Day, a rather inauspicious date we felt!

We had the most marvellous experiences that year. Many friends and family came from Canada and Australia to visit; we joined the local golf club; revelled in the laid-back lifestyle of our local town, Kenmare, where the shops didn't open until ten in the morning and banks and most shops closed for lunch. We made some life-long friends over long gossipy lunches at the local pubs, hiked and cycled and enjoyed Irish coffee at Kate Kearney's cottage. As an artist I painted a series of these Irish scenes and held a successful show at the famous local Kenmare Hotel, with all proceeds going to World Vision. My husband was keen on purchasing one of these cottages to restore and indeed it was very tempting, but I suggested it wasn't practicable having our children in Canada, our lives becoming settled in Australia and also owning an Irish cottage!

Home in Australia once again, we collected the dog and settled back into an easy lifestyle until one day we read a newspaper advertisement about an historic property for sale on the south coast. We fell in love with it and much to our amazement, the following weekend we were the successful bidders at auction! Heavens, now what were we going to do with it?

We took over this charming property which had a farmhouse dating back to 1856, a National Trust schoolhouse, a stables block, masses of roses, lavender hedges, a vineyard, olive trees, lawn tennis court and sandstone swimming pool. Did I mention that it accommodated up to twenty guests and we could run it as a bed and breakfast centre, function centre ... or just live in it? I also failed to mention that it needed a lot of tender loving care! However, over the next five years we did all of that and more. We had wonderful family Christmases and our daughter was married from there.

Several years ago I decided to try to wean myself off HRT because of all the health concerns resulting from the Prempro Study. My local doctor said he felt the result was biased because many of the women in the study already had heart conditions and other health problems. He said, 'It's all a bit like Russian roulette and we all have to make our own informed decisions about what we choose to do.' However, I'd been prompted by friends to try maca powder. Grown high in the Andean mountains of Peru it's been used for 10,000 years to balance the hormones in both men and women, improve PMS, support menopausal health, enhance libido, increase energy, regulate hormonal secretion, improve memory, fight depression, and much more! The powder is mixed into a fruit juice or milk drink and taken daily. I decided to be brave and stopped taking HRT to give maca my best shot. I took it faithfully for six months. Hot flushes and night sweats increased and I suffered from severe leg cramps. I also gained weight and sometimes had light spotting. Now I'm back on my original HRT, albeit half the original dosage. Doctors do not recommend stopping HRT cold turkey and in hindsight it was not a good idea.

Last year I turned sixty and had a pretty scary experience when I was faced with a 'recall' following my regular mammogram. There was a small lump in my breast and they needed to do an ultrasound to check it out. As I sat in the waiting room, surrounded by about a dozen women, many of them older with daughters or friends accompanying them for support, I wondered just what the next few hours would bring and how it might affect my life. I reflected on how I'd flippantly said that if by taking HRT I gained relief from menopausal symptoms but it shortened my life by a few years, then it would have been worth it ... now I wondered. Fortunately my lump was benign but I was given the warning that 'it could change and to keep an eye on it'.

Maybe this year I'll try coming off HRT again. Surely the symptoms can't go on forever! I've spoken to friends who have ceased taking HRT and have done so successfully without any return of symptoms and others who were experiencing flushes every half hour, forgetfulness, insecurity and on the whole couldn't cope without HRT. I think we are all very different; it's a journey we each have to make for ourselves.

This is my journey. Good luck with yours.

Glenda has heeded the warning about the lump in her breast and thinks seriously about her use of HRT. Her current prescription of Premarin and Provera is at the lowest dose available; lower than any patches.

CONCLUSION

You may be wondering who Sally is, to whom this book is dedi-
cated. Sally and I were friends for thirty-three years. We met in
England while I was doing the obligatory two-year working holiday
after finishing high school. We worked together and kept in touch
until her death in 2004. She could not finish her journey. When I
read the Coroner's Report on her suicide, I shouted, 'Enough!
This book needs to be out there.'

It has taken *guts* for women to tell their stories. A couple of
women wanted to drop out of contributing to the book but
continued, knowing that their experiences could help
another. You may read of an experience similar to yours, or
perhaps your menopause may be only a minor interruption
to your life. Whatever your circumstance I hope that the
women in this book have given you encouragement to be
open, ask questions and share information.

Do not be hard on yourself. Accept that menopause is
a part of life just as there are many other stages of life. Talk
about your experiences. Seek information from all sources,
work out what works for you, whether that be HRT,
herbals and naturals, exercise, life-style changes, counselling, prayer – they are all options.

If necessary adjust your life to allow time for rest. Once

in a while treat yourself to time away from chores and commitments. Go on a weekend retreat or have a picnic with friends. Book a full body massage, have breakfast in bed or walk on the beach and watch the sun set. Do something you haven't done for a long time. Go to the zoo, check out the latest art exhibition or the new museum piece. Buy two tickets to a rock concert and take your son. Go to an open air opera with your daughter. Do something you have never done. Learn meditation, join a walking group or a book club. Form your own menopause club, plant a drought-resistant garden, get physical and learn boxing, buy a massive canvas and paint your masterpiece, write your own menopause story.

And when you look in the mirror and an older face looks back, smile and say hi, and remember everyone around you – everyone – is getting older too.

I hope that you have enjoyed this book. It was written for you. Learn from it, take from it and share it.

Happy menopause!

Debra Vinecombe

USEFUL CONTACTS

The following list gives useful web sites and contact details. Further information and other links on menopause can be obtained through:

www.google.com
Type in: menopause

You can obtain addresses for clinics in your state from the Australasian Menopause Society home page on the internet:
www.menopause.org.au

Or try:
www.managingmenopause.org.au
www.earlymenopause.com
www.menopauseinstitute.com.au
www.menopausecentre.com.au
www.menopause.net.au

The Jean Hailes Foundation, Victoria, for information and pamphlets:
Toll Free: 1800 151 441
www.jeanhailes.org.au

Osteoporosis Australia:
Toll Free: 1800 242 141
www.osteoporosis.org.au

Women's health topics:
www.womhealth.org.au
www.healthinsite.gov.au

Women's Healthline for free confidential answers to your
health concerns:
1300 882 880

Women's Health Statewide:
Toll Free: 1800 182 098

Women's Information Service:
Toll Free: 1800 188 158

SIBLINGS

Brothers and sisters of children with special needs

KATE STROHM

Siblings tells what it is like to grow up with a sister or brother who has a disability or chronic illness. The siblings of children with special needs are often the overlooked ones in families struggling to cope.

Kate Strohm, an experienced health professional and journalist who has a sister with cerebral palsy, bravely shares the story of her journey from confusion and distress to greater understanding and acceptance. She also provides a forum for other siblings to describe their struggles with resentment, guilt, grief and isolation, their fears and also their joys.

Besides giving siblings a voice at last, Kate Strohm also provides strategies that siblings themselves, parents and practitioners can use to support brothers and sisters of children with special needs.

ISBN 978 1 86254 580 9

For more information visit www.wakefieldpress.com.au

AN UNCOMMON DIALOGUE

DEBRA J. DRAKE

'Yes, you got through it,' he said quietly, 'but it shouldn't have happened. No little girl should have to put up with that.'

In a psychiatrist's rooms in Adelaide, Debra Drake begins a journey that she hopes will repair the past. She is 41, scared, and desperate for her life to change. In dialogue with her psychiatrist, she relates a past littered with unsuccessful alternative therapies, failed relationships, and sexual abuse. It becomes increasingly clear that her mother, although aware of the abuse, failed to act to protect her daughters.

An Uncommon Dialogue is a true story. Emotional and at times confronting, it travels between the chaos of the present and the sadness of the past. It grapples with the controversial and fascinating concept of multiple personality disorder and reveals how learning to trust within a challenging therapeutic relationship can restore hope and change a life.

ISBN 978 1 86254 679 0

For more information visit www.wakefieldpress.com.au

ADOPTING
Parents' stories

EDITED BY JANE TURNER GOLDSMITH

'But I do want to have a child, with an innate and deeply ingrained part of my being.'

Adopting a child can be a journey of great joy but the path is never without challenges. In *Adopting*, Australian parents recount their experiences of local and intercountry adoption. We share their hopes and doubts as they make their decision to adopt a child, travel with them across the world, share their apprehension and elation when first meeting their child, and return home to witness their early fumbling times as a new family.

'This is your new mother and father, Madhu was told. He argued. He knew what his parents looked like, and we weren't even the right colour.'

Jane Turner Goldsmith is a psychologist and former panel member of the Australians Aiding Children Adoption Agency in South Australia. Between 2001 and 2004 she interviewed parents wishing to adopt children from overseas. *Adopting* is the outcome of a collaborative project to record and represent the voices of adoptive parents and their families. Jane has published a novel, *Poinciana*, short stories and a novel for children, *Gone Fishing*.

ISBN 978 1 86254 768 1

For more information visit www.wakefieldpress.com.au

SEVENTEEN VOICES
Life and wisdom from inside 'mental illness'

MARIANNE BROUG

We know what the words 'mental illness' mean to psychiatrists or doctors. But who are the real experts? These candid interviews bring 'mental illness' to life from the inside out. This book offers solace and encouragement to people who suffer, but also an intensely personal insight into the experiences and opinions of those who have been labelled as 'mentally ill'.

'People need to listen to our stories, listen to our points of view and have a different understanding of mental illness ... I've often said that mental illness is a condition of society.' – Sarah

'My discovery that many of the great spiritual writers – including Mother Teresa of Calcutta – say that suffering is a gift was a great joy to me ... it hit me between the eyes! It makes it so much easier to accept the road that I've travelled down. Suffering can seem to be so negative yet it can, if we allow it, produce in our Being the positive gift of compassion. Compassion doesn't come out of thin air.' – John

'At the clinic I hear people talking about integrating people with "mental illness" into society, but by definition of what they have done, they have made that impossible. They label you as "mentally ill", and then push you back into a society that thinks, Oh my god, "mental illness"!' – Cheryl

'The media portray the "mentally ill" as violent. But the truth is that we'd much rather kill ourselves than anybody else. I apologise to an ant or a spider if I kill it. I don't want to hurt anybody or anything.' – Linda

ISBN 978 1 86254 801 5

For more information visit www.wakefieldpress.com.au

Wakefield Press is an independent publishing and
distribution company based in Adelaide, South Australia.
We love good stories and publish beautiful books.
To see our full range of titles, please visit our website at
www.wakefieldpress.com.au.